LABORATORY WORKBOOK IN
Diagnostic Microbiology

LABORATORY WORKBOOK IN
Diagnostic Microbiology

Edited by

Connie R. Mahon, MS, MT(ASCP)
Department of Clinical Laboratory Sciences
The University of Texas Health Science Center at San Antonio
San Antonio, Texas

George Manuselis, Jr., MA, MT(ASCP)
Medical Technology Program
The Ohio State University
Columbus, Ohio

W.B. SAUNDERS COMPANY
A Division of Harcourt Brace & Company
Philadelphia London Toronto Montreal Sydney Tokyo

W.B. Saunders Company
A Division of Harcourt Brace & Company

The Curtis Center
Independence Square West
Philadelphia, Pennsylvania 19106

Laboratory Workbook in Diagnostic Microbiology   ISBN 0–7216–4029–X

Printed in the United States of America.

Last digit is the print number: 9   8   7   6   5   4   3   2   1

Contributors

SHIRLEY ADAMS, MS, SM(ASCP), CLS
Adjunct Faculty, Greenville Technical College; Medical Technologist II, Greenville Memorial Medical Center, Greenville, South Carolina

PATRICIA K. HARGRAVE, PhD
Assistant Professor, Department of Medical Technology, School of Allied Health, University of Kansas Medical Center, Kansas City, Kansas

Preface

One of the major challenges for clinical laboratory science, clinical laboratory technology, and clinical microbiology students when interpreting primary cultures of clinical samples is to be able to distinguish significant isolates from those that occur as normal colonizers at a particular body site. Students are frequently amazed, during their clinical rotation in microbiology, when they discover that cultures of clinical samples do not always produce single isolates or "pure cultures." Hence, this laboratory workbook is designed to prepare students for their clinical rotation or practicum in clinical microbiology.

Laboratory Workbook in Diagnostic Microbiology has been written to be used in conjunction with our *Textbook of Diagnostic Microbiology.* This laboratory manual consists of three major units:

I: *Laboratory Procedures in Clinical Microbiology.* This unit provides general information and guidelines on laboratory safety; specimen collection, processing, and transport; and smear preparation and specimen inoculation techniques. Also included are exercises for students to develop proficiency in the preparation of smears for Gram stain and in microscopic examination of stained smears. Students are shown how proper interpretation of microscopic morphology along with the description of colonial morphology is used to presumptively identify an unknown isolate. Students are encouraged to illustrate the microscopic morphology of representative organisms and to describe the colonial characteristics of known organisms.

II: *Identification of Infectious Agents.* This unit helps the student to develop confidence and competency in recognizing and identifying microorganisms by reinforcing and applying previously acquired skills, specifically, the skill of utilizing microscopic and colonial morphology to presumptively identify unknown isolates, learned in Unit I.

Selected fungal species are illustrated and discussed; however, because of the biohazardous nature of fungal agents, we do not feel that it is appropriate to perform fungal cultures in the student laboratory *unless* students work under biohazard safety cabinets and with direct supervision. Similarly, mycobacterial smears and cultures are for demonstration purposes only.

III: *Laboratory Diagnosis of Infectious Diseases.* In this unit, the student is introduced to antimicrobial susceptibility procedures and interpretation. Special methods may be either performed by students or demonstrated by the instructor. Exercises are provided for students to practice plate reading and culture interpretation using clinical samples.

Each topic in each unit of *Laboratory Workbook in Diagnostic Microbiology* consists of a set of objectives, a description of the organism or concept to be studied, and laboratory exercises to accomplish the objectives. At the end of each major group of organisms, exercises to work up unknown organisms are provided.

Laboratory Workbook in Diagnostic Microbiology uses the building-block approach, similar to that used in *Textbook of Diagnostic Microbiology,* to present this voluminous material. In addition, it provides a practical approach to identifying clinically significant isolates by using identification schema and networks based on the microscopic and colonial morphology and the source of the isolate. This approach allows students to apply their previously acquired knowledge of diagnostic microbiology and to decide which tests are appropriate to perform to identify an unknown isolate. By using clinical samples as unknowns, students get the opportunity to work up "mixed cultures." This allows them to develop the skills needed to select the organisms that require complete identification because of their potential significance as pathogens at a particular body site.

Because of the biohazardous nature of certain organisms, such as *Mycobacterium tuberculosis, Bacillus anthracis,* and fungi, we suggest that the study of extremely pathogenic organisms be restricted to the use of properly preserved microscopic slides to demonstrate the characteristics of these organisms.

We have selected organisms for laboratory exercises that should demonstrate and represent positive and negative biochemical test reactions. We have also limited the scope of the organisms to those that are commonly encountered in the clinical laboratory. Certainly other organisms that represent similar reactions may be used, and the selection is left to the discretion of the laboratory instructor.

The appendices contain selected media, reagents, and stains that are commonly used. The principles, ingredients, preparation, and interpretation of reactions are included as a resource for the students.

Everyone has a different way of teaching a microbiology laboratory. Finding the perfect laboratory workbook that fully satisfies everyone's needs has been a challenge to most of us who teach in clinical laboratory science programs. *Laboratory Workbook in Diagnostic Microbiology* does not fulfill all those needs; however, we have incorporated into this workbook many suggestions made by students over our many years of teaching. It is our intent to make teaching and learning diagnostic microbiology fun, yet challenging. We therefore would be delighted to hear from users of *Laboratory Workbook in Diagnostic Microbiology* with their suggestions and comments. Until then, we hope that our efforts to prepare students for their practice have served their purpose.

CONNIE R. MAHON MS, MT(ASCP)
GEORGE MANUSELIS, JR., MA, MT(ASCP)

Contents

APPENDICES

Laboratory Procedures in Clinical Microbiology

CHAPTER 1

Safety Procedures in the Clinical Microbiology Laboratory

It is difficult to quantitate the risk of working with an infectious agent in the laboratory. Risk to an individual increases with the frequency and level of contact with the agent. It is therefore important that the laboratory develop and institute a safety program that effectively minimizes overt laboratory-associated hazards to all who have direct or indirect exposure to such hazards. The following information is provided as guidelines for a clinical laboratory. Although most practices also apply to this student laboratory, there may be several that do not apply.

SPECIAL PRECAUTIONS

All personnel working with infectious agents should observe the appropriate safety precautions.

Protective Clothing

1. The following shall be worn while working in the clinical microbiology laboratory:
   - Laboratory coat
   - Disposable gloves
2. If laboratory clothing becomes contaminated with any organism, it should be autoclaved immediately before reusing.
3. Remove protective clothing before leaving the laboratory area.
4. If disposable laboratory coats are not used, laboratory coats should be laundered on a frequent basis.

Handling Specimens

1. Handle all specimens with care.
2. Reject grossly contaminated specimens.
3. Wipe the work area with disinfectant at the beginning and at the end of each laboratory session.
4. If a specimen container is spilled or broken, cover the area with paper towels and flood with disinfectant. Allow disinfectant to stand at least 15 minutes before cleaning the area.
5. Open the specimen container only at the time of inoculation. Do not open a series of containers and leave the lids open.

6. Perform all work over practive sheets. A container of disinfectant must be close at hand.

Disposal of Contaminated Materials

1. Place all used media, swabs, specimens, and other contaminated articles in the biohazard containers.
   - Culture plates and other contaminated paper materials are discarded into plastic double biohazard bags.
   - Bags should be changed when half full.
2. Pipettes and other glass materials are discarded into the plastic biohazard containers.
3. Report any breakage of bags or leakage of containers to the instructors at once for instructions on procedures for safe cleanup.

Other Laboratory Practices

1. Scrub hands thoroughly with soap and water before leaving the laboratory.
2. *Do not* eat, drink, or apply cosmetics in the laboratory.
3. *Do not* mouth pipette under any circumstances.
4. Immediately report all accidents involving injury or infectious aerosols.
5. When working with extremely infectious or highly virulent materials, extreme care should be exercised.
   - Containers should be opened and processed *only* under a biologic safety cabinet.
   - The work area should be covered with clean towels soaked in disinfectant.
   - Protective clothing, including gown, gloves, and mask, should be worn.
   - Individuals processing materials suspected of containing organisms listed as follows should observe all safety precautions and remain isolated in the room until all procedures are completed.
     Mycobacterium tuberculosis
     Brucella sp
     Francisella tularensis
     Pseudomonas pseudomallei
     Yersinia pestis
     Vibrio cholerae
   - Follow all decontamination procedures before leaving the laboratory.

Biologic Safety Cabinet

A biologic safety cabinet encloses a work area to prevent workers from being exposed to infectious agents. A high-efficiency particulate air (HEPA) filter removes most particles from the air that passes into the cabinet and around the material within. Perform all processing of clinical specimens for microbiologic studies in the biologic safety cabinet.

The classification of cabinets is based on the degree of biologic containment they perform.

1. Class I—sterilizes the air to be exhausted.

2. Class II—also called laminar flow, sterilizes air that flows over the infectious material and also the air to be exhausted. Most hospital laboratories use a class II biologic safety cabinet.

3. Class III—sterilizes the air coming into and going out of the cabinet. Because the cabinet is completely enclosed, it offers the most protection to the worker. The infectious material is handled with rubber gloves that are attached and sealed to the cabinet

CHAPTER 2

Procedures for Handling Clinical Specimens for Microbiologic Examination

The proper diagnosis of a bacterial infection depends on the close communication between the microbiologist and the clinician. The clinician should provide a clinical diagnosis that may lead the microbiologist to the isolation and identification of the causative agent. The microbiologist is responsible for providing methods and procedures that demonstrate the probable agent. The microbiologist must also establish procedures for rapid diagnosis and presumptive identification of causative bacterial agents. These procedures may include direct examination or antigen detection using several methods.

The specimen submitted to the laboratory is the primary connection between the patient, clinician, and microbiologist. Failure to choose, transport, and process the clinical sample appropriately may lead to establishing a wrong diagnosis or failing to isolate the true causative agent of the disease.

Hence, the microbiologist must establish procedures for proper specimen collection, preservation, and transport to the laboratory. The technologist must process the samples as they are received and evaluate them for suitability and integrity. This chapter covers several procedures for handling clinical specimens for microbiologic examinations, including:

- Specimen collection, transport, and processing
- Smear preparation, staining, and interpretation
- Media selection for cultivation
- Procedures for inoculation of media for colony isolation and semiquantitation

▓▓▓▓ O B J E C T I V E S

1. Describe proper specimen collection procedures and appropriate transport medium when necessary for each of the following clinical samples:

   - Urine clean catch
   - Sputum
   - Abscess
   - Cervical exudate
   - Stool

2. Prepare and stain smears from different types of clinical material or cultures of microorganisms in liquid or solid media.

3. Discuss the principle of Gram stain procedure including the purpose of each reagent.

4. Perform the Gram stain procedure and obtain expected results.

5. Describe the expected appearance of gram-positive and gram-negative bacteria.

6. Interpret and report bacterial smears including quantitation of white blood count and epithelial cells.

7. Describe the microscopic morphology of the organisms found.

8. Evaluate the quality of clinical samples received to determine their suitability for culture.

9. Inoculate various culture media to achieve isolated bacterial colonies and to presumptively identify the isolates.

10. Select appropriate culture media for cultivation of significant organisms from clinical materials.

SPECIMEN COLLECTION, TRANSPORT, AND PROCESSING

Proper specimen collection, transport, and processing are essential elements in the correct diagnosis and proper interpretation of bacterial culture results. Clinical samples improperly collected may provide information that is misleading with regards to the cause of the disease. Specimens received in the laboratory that are not properly preserved or are not in transport media may provide nonviable organisms and yield sterile cultures. Various transport media are available to minimize the effects of delay between specimen collection and processing. These transport media must be used to prevent drying, maintain the proper environment for the organism, and minimize growth of contaminating normal flora.

Guidelines for Specimen Collection

1. Throat and nasopharynx. Most often throat cultures are obtained to recover group A β-hemolytic streptococcus. To obtain the sample for throat culture, ask the patient to open the mouth wide, take a deep breath, and say an "ahh." Using a tongue blade, depress the tongue gently and touch the posterior pharynx gently with a swab, swabbing the tonsillar pillars and mucosa.

2. Sputum and lower respiratory tract. Sputum and lower respiratory secretions are usually contaminated with organisms that inhabit the upper respiratory tract. The first morning deep coughed-up specimen is preferred. Other methods of collecting respiratory specimens are:

   - Induced with nebulized saline through a positive-pressure respirator apparatus
   - Transtracheal aspiration—performed when anaerobic pulmonary infection is suspected and routine cultures are negative
   - Bronchoscopy sample—also contaminated with upper respiratory flora

3. Urine cultures require clean-catch samples. Other procedures used are suprapubic aspiration and catheterization.

4. Wounds are usually contaminated with normal skin flora. Cleanse around the surface of cutaneous wounds with 70% alcohol. If possible, aspirate the purulent material from the infected site.

5. Stool samples should be examined and cultured as soon as possible. As the specimen cools off, the pH drop is sufficient to inhibit most *Shigella* sp and some *Salmonella* strains.

6. Cerebrospinal fluid is obtained by lumbar spinal puncture. A long spinal needle is inserted between the third and fourth lumbar vertebrae and cerebro-

spinal fluid flows under pressure. Three to four tubes are usually collected for various procedures. Do not refrigerate.

7. Eye, ear, and sinus. Suppurative material from an infected eye should be collected from the lower cul-de-sac. Smear for Gram stain should always be made. Ear cultures are best collected by an otolaryngologist in cases of a perforated eardrum. The external ear does not yield any significant culture results. Aspiration technique is applied for maxillary and frontal sinuses for isolation of both aerobic and anaerobic organisms in chronic sinusitis.

8. Blood. Several factors affect the successful isolation of causative agents of bacteremia:

- Use of aseptic technique imperative
- Number and timing of collection (two to three per 24 hours)
- Volume (at least 10 mL)
- Culture medium used—must contain sodium polyanethol sulfonate (SPS), which is an anticoagulant; also inhibits complement and phagocytosis and inactivates most therapeutic concentration of aminoglycosides

9. Tissues/biopsy specimens. Bone marrow is inoculated into blood culture bottles. Tissues and biopsy samples are ground and inoculated into either a supplemented broth culture medium or blood culture medium.

Guidelines for Specimen Transport and Processing

Clinical samples must be maintained as near their original state as possible. The standard time limit is 2 hours from the time the sample is collected. Transport medium must be used whenever a delay in processing is expected.

Guidelines for Specimen Processing

Clinical specimens received in the microbiology laboratory must be evaluated visually and microscopically to determine suitability. Criteria as to when to reject a clinical sample submitted to the laboratory must be established within the laboratory.

Examine samples to make sure that:

The sample is properly collected.
It is in an appropriate container.
There is sufficient quantity.
There has been no excessive time delay.

SMEAR PREPARATION, STAINING, AND INTERPRETATION

The significance of microscopic examination cannot be overemphasized. It provides information that leads to the proper identification of the microorganism. Direct examination of stained preparations of clinical material is used to determine whether the sample is appropriately collected and is representative of the infection site. This examination may also give a presumptive diagnosis when the presence of bacteria and white blood cells is observed. Some bacterial species demonstrate characteristic morphology that also provides an immediate preliminary identification.

Direct Smears

These are smears prepared directly from the clinical specimen at smear preparation. Such a smear is useful for several reasons:

- Findings in the direct smear may confirm or reject a diagnosis. This information may also differentiate between two possible diagnoses and allow immediate initiation of proper treatment on the same day the specimen is received in the laboratory.
- The number and type of cells present on the direct smear may help establish a diagnosis or interpret the results of the culture. The direct smear examination allows visualization of the predominating type of organism.
- Occasionally an organism that does not appear in the culture is seen in the direct smear. There are several possible explanations for this:
  a. The organism is one that grows slowly. It will appear if the culture is held longer.
  b. The patient has received sufficient treatment (usually antibiotics) to prevent the growth of the organism.
  c. The specimen had stood too long before the culture was inoculated. Some organisms die if left too long at room temperature or allowed to dry.
  d. The organism requires a special medium or some special condition that was not provided in the culture.

Preparation of Smears

Direct Smears

Only one smear should be put on each slide. Use slides with frosted ends so that each slide can be fully identified. A lead pencil can be used for slide identification.

1. Prepare only one smear on each slide.
2. Label with a lead pencil the slides with frosted ends so that each slide can be fully identified.
3. When preparing a smear from:

   a. Swabs
      - When swabs are used to prepare the smear, roll the swab across the slide to avoid destruction of cellular entities (Fig. 2–1).
   b. Concentrated centrifuged specimens
      - Prepare smears of concentrated centrifuged specimens by using a sterile, rubber-bulbed Pasteur pipette (Fig. 2–2A).
      - Place a drop on the slide. Spread the drop to an even film with the tip of the pipette (Fig. 2–2B).

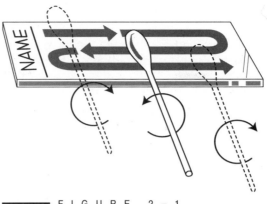
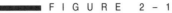

■■■ F I G U R E   2 - 1

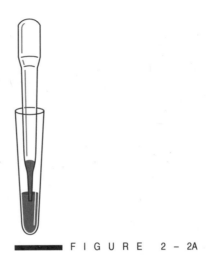

■■■ F I G U R E   2 - 2A

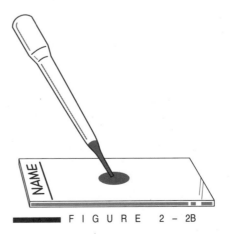

■■■ F I G U R E   2 - 2B

Smears from Cultures (Subculture Smears)

Most routine staining procedures involve the preparation of a smear from bacterial cultures. This is done by spreading a thin film of bacteria on the surface of a clean glass slide.

It is more economical of both time and materials to make several smears on one slide. This will not lead to confusion if you develop a routine and follow it each time.

1. Use plain slides without frosted ends. Leave an area at the left end of the slide for a number or other identification. Mark the slide into three small squares with a glass-marking pencil. Turn the slide over so that the pencil marks are down (Fig. 2–3A).

2. On a sheet of paper, record the number of the slide. Below, list the numbers 1 through 3. As you make smears, record the source of each opposite the corresponding number.

Smears from Liquid Media

Place a loopful of culture in the square. Unless growth is exceptionally heavy, do not spread (Fig. 2–3B).

Smears from Solid Media

Place a small drop of water in the square (Fig. 2–4A). In this, emulsify a colony or a portion of a colony (Fig. 2–4B). Unless the colony is quite tiny, it

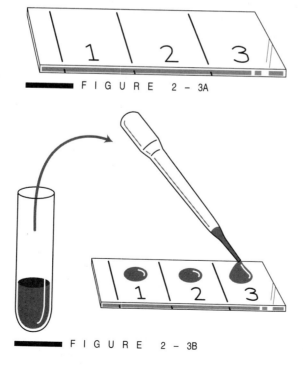

■■■■ F I G U R E   2 – 3A

■■■■ F I G U R E   2 – 3B

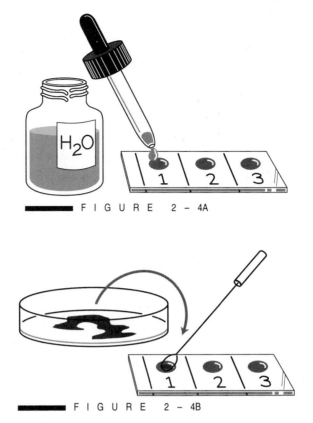

■■■■ F I G U R E   2 – 4A

■■■■ F I G U R E   2 – 4B

is usually best to spread this emulsion over the entire area. Allow the smears to air-dry.

Precautions

1. Be especially careful that material in one square does not overflow or splatter into another square.

2. Try to make all the smears on one side as nearly the same thickness as is practical. If some are much heavier than others, great care must be used in destaining.

3. When destaining the slide, you will find that the water used to wash off the iodine tends to "pile up" at the lower end of the slide. This can be removed by touching the corner of the slide to the staining rack. If this water is not removed, it may dilute the acetone, which slows the destaining process in this area.

4. The pencil marks sometimes wash off during staining. If you have more than one slide, be sure to repair the identifying number as soon as the slide is stained. If you always follow the same system when dividing the slide into squares, you will be able to find individual smears even though the pencil marks have washed off.

GRAM STAIN PROCEDURE

A. Principle of Procedure

Bacteriologists use the Gram stain (perfected by the Danish bacteriologist Christian Gram) to observe the cellular morphology of most organisms. The cells are stained with a basic dye (crystal violet) that is taken up in similar amounts by all bacteria. The slides are then treated with an iodine–potassium iodide mixture to fix (mordant) the stain, washed with acetone alcohol, and finally counterstained with a paler dye of different color (safranin). Gram-positive organisms retain the initial violet stain, whereas gram-negative organisms are decolorized by the organic solvent and hence show the counterstain.

B. Reagents

Staining reagents are available commercially.

1. Crystal violet (Hucker modification)
   - Ready to use
   - Store at 15 to 30°C
2. Gram iodine solution
   - Store at 15 to 30°C
3. Decolorizer
   - Ready to use
   - Store at 15 to 30°C
4. Safranin
   - Ready to use
   - Store at 15 to 30°C

C. Quality Control

- *Staphylococcus aureus* = Gram positive
- *Escherichia coli* = Gram negative

1. If expected results are not obtained, repeat the procedure using fresh reagents.
2. If results are still out of control, notify the instructor and record action taken in the *out of control section* of the *Quality Control log sheets.*

D. Procedure

1. Heat-fix slides by holding the slide against the front of the incinerator. An alternative method is fixing the slides with 50 to 70% methanol.
2. Cover the prepared slide with crystal violet; stain for 1 minute.
3. Pour off stain and wash with running tap water.
4. Mordant with Gram iodine for about 1 minute.
5. Rinse in running water and shake off excess water.
6. Decolorize rapidly with acetone-alcohol solution; this may take as little as 5 seconds or up to 20 seconds depending on the thickness of the smear.
7. Remove excess decolorizer with a gentle flow of water.
8. Counterstain with safranin for about 10 to 12 seconds.
9. Wash briefly with tap water, blot dry, and examine the smear microscopically under oil immersion objective.

E. Expected results

1. Gram-positive organisms are blue.
2. Gram-negative organisms are red.

INTERPRETATION AND REPORTING OF BACTERIAL SMEARS

1. When examining a direct smear, first look for cells: epithelial cells, red blood cells, or white blood cells. Red blood cells may stain faintly but are usually recognizable. On Gram-stained smear, the nucleus of white blood cells should appear red. The white cells can be differentiated only into polymorphonuclear cells and mononuclear cells. No further differentiation should be attempted with this stain. The most frequently seen cell is a "poly" that has begun to disintegrate and is called a "pus" cell. Report the kind of cells present, if any, and the approximate number.

2. Look for microorganisms. Enumerate the number of polymorphonuclear cells and the number of organisms found, indicating:

    a. Many . . . . (4+) . . . . 10–20/oil immersion field
    b. Moderate . . . .(3+) . . . . 6–10/oil immersion field
    c. Few . . . . (2+) . . . . 3–5/oil immersion field
    d. Rare . . . . (1+) . . . . less than 10 seen on entire smear
3. Examine the organisms present and describe the organisms as follows:
    a. Gram stain reaction
    b. Shape
    c. Characteristic morphology or arrangement:
- Gram-positive or gram-negative
- Coccus, bacilli, spirochete, curved-rod
- Large or small, single, in pairs, clusters, or chains
- Pleomorphic, coccobacillary or diphtheroid, if applicable
- If spores are present, note location (terminal or subterminal), shape (oval or round), and if spores swell the cells

Report the approximate number of each organism observed. A typical direct smear report might read:

3+ epithelial cells
1+ red blood cells
4+ gram-negative rods
2+ gram-positive cocci in pairs

PROCEDURES FOR SELECTION, INOCULATION, AND INITIAL INTERPRETATION OF PRIMARY MEDIA

Selection of Primary Media

Isolation of the infecting agent in culture is still the most sensitive and specific means of laboratory diagnosis of infectious diseases. Most bacteria can be cultivated in vitro using artificial culture media. The primary media selected for cultivation of organisms depend on the suspected causative agent from a particular clinical sample. Clinical microbiology laboratories use a wide variety of growth media for isolation of commonly encountered bacterial agents. In addition, laboratories provide media for isolation of unusual and fastidious organisms that require special nutrients on request.

There are several types of culture media used for specific purposes. These media are classified as: nutrient, selective, and differential or indicator. A *nutrient* medium is used primarily to satisfy the growth requirements of bacteria. This medium supports the growth of most nonfastidious organisms. For other pathogens that require special nutrients for growth, vitamins, salts, and body fluids may be added to the nutrient base.

Selective media are used when specific significant organisms are to be isolated. Chemical dyes or antimicrobials are added to the medium to inhibit contaminating organisms but not the suspected agent. *Indicator* or *differential* media are designed to demonstrate certain diagnostic features of specific pathogens. The medium contains an indicator system, such as a pH indicator, and a carbohydrate, which shows color change of the colony when the carbohydrate is used. *Broth* medium is used as enrichment medium to allow small numbers of organisms to grow.

Table 2–1 lists the most common sources of clinical samples and the suggested primary plating media for cultivation of significant organisms.

■■■ T A B L E   2 – 1
PRIMARY PLATING MEDIA FOR COMMON CLINICAL SAMPLES

Specimen	Routine Media	Temperature/Atmosphere
Throat	BAP	35°C, CO_2
Sputum	BAP, MaC, Choc	35°C, CO_2
Urine	BAP, MaC	35°C
Stool/rectal	BAP, MaC, HE, Sel F	35°C
Cerebrospinal fluid, other body fluids	MaC, Thio, BAP, Choc	35°C, CO_2
Cervical, vaginal, urethral	BAP, TM, MaC, Thio broth	35°C, CO_2
Abscess, wounds	BAP, Choc, MaC, ana BAP, Thio broth	35°C, CO_2
Eye, ear	BAP, Choc, MaC, Thio broth	35°C, CO_2
Skin, pustules	BAP, Choc, MaC, Thio broth	35°C, CO_2

Inoculation Techniques

There are several methods of inoculating culture media. The method used depends on its purposes.

The first method described is used primarily to obtain well-isolated colonies on primary isolation media. The second technique described is used to estimate semiquantitatively bacterial concentration in the urine samples.

■■■ **PROCEDURES**

A. Inoculation to Achieve Isolation of Bacterial Colonies (Fig. 2–5)

1. Apply a portion of specimen to an area near the periphery of the plate.
2. With a bacteriologic loop, distribute the specimen across the agar by spreading the specimen back and forth over the surface of about one quarter of the plate.
3. After the first quadrant has been inoculated, sterilize the loop by flaming it over a Bunsen burner or incinerator; let it cool.

■■■ F I G U R E   2 – 5

4. Turn the plate 90 degrees. Touch the original inoculum with the first cross-streaks.
5. Continue to inoculate the surface of the agar. Avoid touching the original inoculum.
6. When another quarter of the plate is covered, turn the plate another 90 degrees, and the process is repeated.

B. Streaking with a Calibrated Loop to Estimate Bacterial Concentration in the Urine (Fig. 2–6)

1. Pick up a loopful of fluid and deposit it at the top of the blood agar plate. Spread the fluid down the entire length of the plate.
2. Without flaming the loop, streak back and forth closely across the original streak.

3. Cross-streak to spread the fluid evenly over the entire surface. This pattern is to achieve a total colony count of organisms.

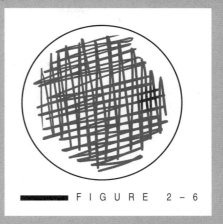

■ F I G U R E   2 – 6

Initial Observation and Interpretation of Primary Cultures

Gross Colony Characteristics

Microbiologists observe the colonial morphology of the organisms isolated on primary cultures after 18 hours of incubation. This initial interpretation provides the microbiologist with information on how to proceed in identifying the isolated organism.

The following are terms commonly used to describe gross colony characteristics:

■■■■■ C O L O N Y   C H A R A C T E R I S T I C S   A N D
D E S C R I P T I O N   O F   B A C T E R I A L   C O L O N I E S

Medium _____
Diameter in mm _____
Color _____
Surface (glistening, dull, other)
Density (opaque, translucent, other)
Consistency (butyrous, viscid, membranous, brittle, other)

	Form
punctiform	irregular
circular	rhizoid

Chart continued on following page

■■■■■■ C O L O N Y   C H A R A C T E R I S T I C S   A N D   D E S C R I P T I O N   O F   B A C T E R I A L   C O L O N I E S

Continued

spindle

filament

flat

Elevation
pulvinate

raised

umbonate

convex

umbilicate

entire

Margin
erose

undulate

filamentous

lobate

curled

Hemolysis on Blood Agar

- α
- β
- Nonhemolytic

Pigment Produced

Odor Produced

Use of Gram Stain and Microscopic Morphology for Preliminary Identification

By observing the colony morphology of the organisms isolated, the microbiologist has a "calculated guess" of the identification of the causative agent. The microbiologist confirms this presumptive identification by studying the microscopic characteristics based on Gram stain reaction and cellular morphology. Smears can be made from each different colony type, stained with Gram stain, and examined under the microscope. The microbiologist's evaluation of the stained smear and assessment of the bacterial colonies provide information toward correct identification of the bacteria.

Initial Interpretation of Primary Cultures

1. After 18 to 24 hours of incubation, examine all plates for growth.
2. List the number of different colony types observed from each of the sources.
3. Estimate the amount of each colony type by observing growth at the first, second, third, and fourth quadrant.
4. Describe the gross colony characteristics such as:
   - ■ Color
   - ■ Elevation
   - ■ Density
   - ■ Hemolysis on blood agar plates
5. Prepare a smear and Gram stain each different colony type isolated.
6. Examine under the microscope and observe the microscopic morphology.
7. Record results on the space provided.
8. Semiquantitate the colony count of the organisms recovered from the urine sample by counting the number of colonies present. Then determine the CFU per mL by multiplying the amount of colonies with the amount of urine inoculated on the agar medium.

■■■■■■■■   LABORATORY EXERCISE 1

SMEAR PREPARATION, STAINING, AND INTERPRETATION

Instructions: The following organisms demonstrate the variation in shape and arrangement of certain bacterial species.

Prepared Smears

1. Gram stain the prepared smears of the following organisms:
   - *Staphylococcus aureus*
   - Group A streptococcus
   - *Neisseria* sp
   - Diphtheroids
   - *Bacillus* sp
   - *Streptococcus pneumoniae*
   - *Candida* sp
   - *Haemophilus* sp
   - *Escherichia coli*
   - *Pseudomonas* sp

2. Observe and describe the microscopic morphology of each organism indicating the:
   - Gram stain reaction
   - Shape
   - Arrangement

   Include any variations in shape and size.

3. Sketch a few cells from each smear demonstrating the characteristic morphology.

■■■■■■■   LABORATORY WORKSHEET 1

SMEAR PREPARATION, STAINING, AND INTERPRETATION

Sketch a few cells demonstrating the characteristic morphology.

Prepared Smears

Staphylococcus aureus
Gram stain: _____
Morphology: _____
_____
_____

Streptococcus pneumoniae
Gram stain: _____
Morphology: _____
_____
_____

Group A streptococcus
Gram stain: _____
Morphology: _____
_____
_____

Candida sp
Gram stain: _____
Morphology: _____
_____
_____

Worksheet continued on following page

■■■■■■■■ LABORATORY WORKSHEET 1 *Continued*

SMEAR PREPARATION, STAINING, AND INTERPRETATION

Neisseria sp
Gram stain: _____
Morphology: _____
_____
_____

Haemophilus sp
Gram stain: _____
Morphology: _____
_____
_____

Diphtheroid
Gram stain: _____
Morphology: _____
_____
_____

Bacillus sp
Gram stain: _____
Morphology: _____
_____
_____

Escherichia coli
Gram stain: _____
Morphology: _____
_____
_____

Pseudomonas sp
Gram stain: _____
Morphology: _____
_____
_____

LABORATORY EXERCISE 2

SMEAR PREPARATION, STAINING, AND INTERPRETATION

Instructions:

1. Prepare smears from the following:

   ■ Broth medium
   ■ Solid medium

2. Prepare a direct smear from a clinical sample, i.e., sputum exudate.
3. Gram stain the smears prepared from the above-mentioned sources.
4. Study and evaluate the smears as described in the previous procedures.
5. Sketch a few cells from the smears.

6. Describe the morphology of the organisms observed indicating the:

   ■ Gram stain reaction
   ■ Shape
   ■ Arrangement

7. Indicate the presence of:

   ■ White blood cells
   ■ Red blood cells
   ■ Epithelial cells

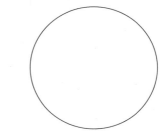

Source
Gram stain reaction: _____
Morphology: _____
_____

Source
Gram stain reaction: _____
Morphology: _____
_____

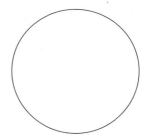

Source: _____
_____
Observation: _____
_____

Source: _____
_____
Observation: _____
_____

Exercise continued on following page

LABORATORY EXERCISE 2 *Continued*

Source: _____

_____

_____

Observation: _____

_____

Source: _____

_____

_____

Observation: _____

_____

■■■■■■■ LABORATORY EXERCISE 3

A. INOCULATION OF CULTURE MEDIA

Instructions:

1. Using Table 2–1 as a guideline, inoculate the clinical samples on the appropriate media.
2. Incubate the inoculated media at the appropriate temperature and environmental condition.
3. Inoculate a urine sample on the appropriate media using the inoculation technique for semiquantitation.
4. Incubate the inoculated media at 37°C for 18 to 24 hours.

███████   LABORATORY WORKSHEET 3

B. Initial Interpretation of Primary Cultures

Student Name _____   Date performed _____
Specimen source: Date completed _____

List the number of different colony types observed.

Number of colony types:

Microscopic Morphology

Isolate 1
Gram stain: _____

Isolate 2
Gram stain: _____

███████   C O L O N I A L   M O R P H O L O G Y

Colony Description	BAP Isolate		MacConkey Isolate	
	1	2	1	2
Growth				
Color				
Density				
Hemolysis				
Elevation				

Note: Smears for Gram stain should only be prepared from a nonselective medium such as BAP.

Worksheet continued on opposite page

■■■■■■■ LABORATORY WORKSHEET 3 *Continued*

Specimen Source:
Microscopic Morphology

Isolate 1
Gram stain: _____

Isolate 2
Gram stain: _____

■■■■■ C O L O N I A L   M O R P H O L O G Y

Colony Description	BAP Isolate		MacConkey Isolate	
	1	*2*	*1*	*2*
Growth				
Color				
Density				
Hemolysis				
Elevation				

Worksheet continued on following page

■■■■■■   LABORATORY WORKSHEET 3 *Continued*

Microscopic Morphology

Isolate 1
Gram stain: _____

Isolate 2
Gram stain: _____

■■■■■ S P E C I M E N   S O U R C E :   U R I N E
Colony count: _____

Colony Description	BAP Isolate		MacConkey Isolate	
	1	*2*	*1*	*2*
Growth				
Color				
Density				
Hemolysis				
Elevation				

CHAPTER *3*

Quality Control in Microbiology

A well-organized, comprehensive quality control program serves to document that the monitoring of procedures, instruments, and products has been performed. These written records should contain actual observations, expected results, and the action taken if the results are outside acceptable limits. Quality control and quality assurance procedures in microbiology are fully described in Chapter 4, *Textbook of Diagnostic Microbiology.*

■■■■■ O B J E C T I V E S

1. Monitor equipment performance such as:

   - Temperature
   - Atmospheric condition
   - Other function checks

2. Document acceptable performance of all reagents, stains, and antisera used in the laboratory.

3. Check sterility and performance of all prepared media by testing with appropriate control organisms.

4. Describe the expected performance results on the following culture media when tested with appropriate control organisms:

   - Sheep blood agar
   - MacConkey agar
   - Eosin–methylene blue agar
   - Thioglycollate medium
   - Chocolate agar
   - Hektoen agar
   - Thayer-Martin agar
   - TSI agar

PROCEDURES THAT MUST BE PERFORMED AT STATED TIME INTERVALS

General Guidelines

- All equipment used in the laboratory must be kept clean and in good condition.
- Instrument maintenance should include temperature and performance checks whenever applicable.
- Proper care of microscopes is essential to ensure adequate resolution when reading smears.

Equipment Check

1. Check the temperature for each incubator, water bath, refrigerator, and freezer at the beginning of each work day and record on the log sheet.

2. Check autoclave once a week using spore strips. Record results on the appropriate log sheet.

3. Anaerobic and CO_2 Systems—BBL Gas Pak Indicator (Cockeysville, MD) (methylene blue) is used in the anaerobe jar to check anaerobiasis. In addition, a culture of *Clostridium* species is placed in the Gas Pak system once a week to ensure suitable conditions to support the growth of anaerobes.

4. Cultures of *Neisseria gonorrhoeae* and *Haemophilus influenzae* are maintained in the CO_2 jar to ensure proper conditions to support the growth of fastidious organisms.

Media, Reagents, and Stains

Stock cultures of organisms for use in monitoring media performance must be maintained in the clinical microbiology laboratory.

1. Prepared media—upon receipt, label each carton received from manufacturer with date received. An expiration date is marked on each plate and tube of medium. Keep a log of the dates received, lot numbers, and expiration dates of all media coming into the laboratory.

2. Performance testing:

   a. Check for sterility:
   ■ Incubate 10% of all tube and plate media received at 35°C overnight.
   b. Performance:
   ■ Check one plate or tube from each new lot number received with appropriate organisms for proper positive and negative reactions.
   ■ Record results.
   ■ Check at monthly intervals any lot number that remains a month or longer or any media giving questionable results.
   ■ Record results on the quality control log sheets.

Chemicals, Stains, and Reagents

The following quality control procedures must be performed when indicated in the laboratory procedure.

1. Label all chemicals with date received, date placed in service, and expiration date.

2. Label all reagents and stains with:

   ■ Date prepared
   ■ Strength
   ■ Expiration date
   ■ Initials of person preparing

3. Check all reagents and stains with a known positive and negative control each day the reagent or stain is used.

4. Record all results on the appropriate log sheets.

Antimicrobial Disks for Susceptibility Testing

1. Include susceptibility tests of *E. coli* ATCC 25922 and *S. aureus* ATCC 25923 each day with the routine batch of antimicrobial susceptibility studies.

2. Measure the zone sizes.

3. Record results on the susceptibility quality control log sheet.

Antisera

1. Label antisera with date received and date opened.

2. Run positive and negative controls each time the serum is used to type an unknown organism.

Note: Any time that results on any quality control procedure do not meet satisfactory requirements the supervisor should be notified, action taken, and the action recorded on the quality control log sheet.

■■■■■■■■ LABORATORY EXERCISE

QUALITY CONTROL

Instructions:

1. Following Table 3–1, inoculate the culture media with the control organisms indicated.

2. Incubate inoculated media in the appropriate temperature and atmosphere.

3. Record all results on the laboratory worksheet.

■■■■■■ T A B L E   3 – 1
PERFORMANCE GUIDELINES FOR MEDIA QUALITY CONTROL

Medium/Temperature, Atmosphere	Control Organisms	Expected Results
Sheep blood	Group A streptococcus	Growth, β-hemolytic
35°C, CO_2	*Streptococcus viridans*	Growth, α-hemolytic
Sheep blood	*Staphylococcus aureus*	Growth, hemolytic
35°C, CO_2	*Staphylococcus epidermidis*	Growth, nonhemolytic
EMB agar	*Escherichia coli*	Growth, metallic sheen
35°C	*Proteus mirabilis*	Growth, colorless
MacConkey	*Pseudomonas aeruginosa*	Growth, colorless
35°C	*E. coli*	Growth, dark pink
	P. mirabilis	Growth, colorless
Hektoen	*E. coli*	Growth, yellow
35°C	*Salmonella* sp	Growth, green with black centers
	P. mirabilis	
Chocolate	*Haemophilus influenzae*	Growth
35°C, CO_2	*Neisseria meningitidis*	Growth
Thayer-Martin	*Neisseria gonorrhoeae*	Growth
35°C, CO_2	*S. epidermidis/Candida* sp	No growth
TSI agar	*E. coli*	A/Ag
35°C	*P. mirabilis*	K/Ag H_2S
	P. aeruginosa	K/K

███████   LABORATORY WORKSHEET

QUALITY CONTROL

Student Name _____   Date performed: _____
                                                       Date completed: _____

Culture Medium	Control Organisms	Results
Sheep blood	Group A streptococcus	
	Streptococcus viridans	
	Staphylococcus aureus	
	Staphylococcus epidermidis	
EMB	Escherichia coli	
	Proteus mirabilis	
MacConkey	E. coli	
	P. mirabilis	
	Pseudomonas aeruginosa	
Hektoen	E. coli	
	Salmonella sp	
	P. mirabilis	
Chocolate	Haemophilus influenzae	
	Neisseria meningitidis	
Thayer-Martin	Neisseria gonorrhoeae	
	S. epidermidis/Candida sp	
TSI	E. coli	
	P. mirabilis	
	P. aeruginosa	

Identification of
Infectious Agents

CHAPTER **4**

Gram-Positive Cocci

This chapter discusses the most commonly encountered gram-positive cocci: *Staphylococcus aureus,* coagulase-negative staphylococci, *Staphylococcus epidermidis, Staphylococcus saprophyticus,* and clinically important streptococci.

▰▰▰ O B J E C T I V E S

1. Perform and interpret correctly each test used to identify staphylococcal species.

2. Differentiate staphylococcal species from other gram-positive cocci.

3. Use the schema in the differentiation and identification of staphylococcal species.

4. Perform the tests appropriate for the identification of the streptococcal species and the expected results for

each. Differentiate the hemolysis produced by each streptococcal group.

5. For each of the tests, describe the principle and list the reagents and quality control procedures used.

6. Given a set of unknowns, correctly identify the organisms present.

7. Describe and differentiate colonial morphology of staphylococcal and streptococcal species.

STAPHYLOCOCCI

Staphylococci belong to the family *Micrococcaceae,* which consists of catalase-positive, facultatively anaerobic, gram-positive cocci that usually appear in clusters and packets. Normally found as inhabitants of the skin and mucous membranes, most species of staphylococci have been associated with a variety of infections. *Staphylococcus aureus* is responsible for skin infections such as boils, carbuncles, and purulent abscesses. Coagulase-negative staphylococci such as *Staphylococcus epidermidis* have been known to be responsible for prosthetic valve infections. *Staphylococcus saprophyticus* is associated with urinary tract infections in women. In addition to staphylococci, micrococci are found as members of the skin flora and are isolated as common contaminants.

Species of staphylococci are differentiated by the coagulase test. Coagulase-producing staphylococcus is identified as *S. aureus.* Those that do not produce coagulase are referred to as *coagulase-negative staphylococci.* Traditionally, glucose fermentation has been used to differentiate coagulase-negative staphylococci from micrococci. More reliable tests may be employed.

On gram-stained smear, staphylococci appear in clusters like bunches of grapes. Staphylococci grow on all the usual noninhibitory laboratory media. These organisms are most often isolated on blood agar. The colonies are round; are at least 1 to 2 mm in diameter; are convex, opaque, glistening, with an entire edge; and are soft or butter-like in consistency. Some varieties are surrounded by zones of hemolysis. The color of the colony varies from an off-white to cream colored to golden yellow.

Many selective media, such as phenylethyl alcohol agar and Columbia Cna, have been developed for the isolation of staphylococci from mixed cultures. Most of these contain an inhibitory substance that prevents the growth of other organisms.

Table 4–1 shows differentiating characteristics between staphylococci and micrococci.

Figures 4–1 and 4–2 are schematic diagrams that show the identification of *Micrococcaceae.* Staphylocoagulase is a substance (possibly an enzyme) produced by potentially pathogenic strains of staphylococci. The amount of coagulase produced in vitro shows no correlation with the severity of the lesion caused by the particular strain. The mode of action of coagulase is not known, although many theories have been advanced. It has been found that purified fibrinogen (which can be clotted by the addition of thrombin) cannot be clotted by staphylocoagulase. This suggests that some other factor is necessary. When plasma is kept in the refrigerator for long periods, there is a progressive loss of coagulability. This loss seems to be due to the loss of this unidentified accessory factor.

Coagulase is not inhibited by hirudin, heparin, dicumarol, or other anticoagulants. Ca^{++} is not required for its action. Heating plasma to 56°C for 4 minutes renders it noncoagulable by staphylocoagulase.

Some human plasmas contain inhibitors to in vitro coagulase activity. This "anticoagulase," however, is slow acting. The addition of coagulase to plasma leads to clotting before the anticoagulase has time to act. Some substances such as sodium azide, streptomycin, erythromycin, and pyocanin inhibit coagulation. It is not clear whether these substances inactivate the coagulase or interfere with its formation. The presence of *Proteus* or hemolytic streptococci may interfere with the reaction.

When citrated plasma is used, false-positive test results may be produced by some gram-negative bacilli and some streptococci, although the clotting agent involved is distinct from staphylocoagulase. It is thought that these bacteria can use citrate in the presence of peptone. This reaction liberates Ca^{++}, which brings about clotting of the plasma. Oxalated or heparinized plasmas are not affected in this way.

■■■■■ T A B L E   4 – 1
IDENTIFICATION OF CLINICALLY SIGNIFICANT MICROCOCCACEAE

Test(s)	Staphylococcus aureus	Staphylococcus epidermidis	Staphylococcus saprophyticus	Micrococcus luteus	Micrococcus roseus	Micrococcus varians
Pigment	Gold-white	White-yellow	White-yellow	Yellow	Pink	Yellow
Hemolysis	+	−	−	−	−	−
Catalase	+	+	+	+	+	−
Coagulase	+	−	−	−	−	−
Novobiocin	S	S	R	S/R	S	R
O-F Glucose	F	F	F(W)	−	O/−	O/−
Mannitol	+	−	+	−	−	−
Nitrate	+	+	+	−	+	+
Phosphatase	+	+	−	−	−	−

F: ferment; O: oxidize; S: susceptible; R: resistant; W: weak.

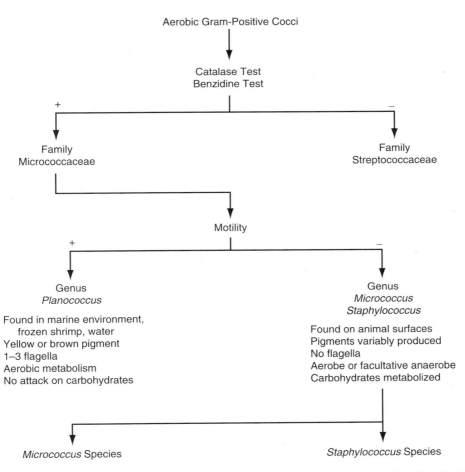

Aerobic Gram-Positive Cocci

Catalase Test
Benzidine Test

+

Family
Micrococcaceae

−

Family
Streptococcaceae

Motility

+

Genus
Planococcus

Found in marine environment,
    frozen shrimp, water
Yellow or brown pigment
1–3 flagella
Aerobic metabolism
No attack on carbohydrates

−

Genus
Micrococcus
Staphylococcus

Found on animal surfaces
Pigments variably produced
No flagella
Aerobe or facultative anaerobe
Carbohydrates metabolized

Micrococcus Species

- G+C content of DNA (moles %) = 66–73
- Teichoic acids in cell wall
- No growth and anaerobic fermentation of glucose
- No anaerobic growth in modified Brewer's
    semisolid thioglycollate medium
- No acid aerobically in glycerol containing 0.4 μg/ml
    of erythromycin
- Resistant to lysostaphin
- Oxidase (DMSO) positive
- Colony size on blood agar at 24 hours = pinpoint
- No growth at 45°C
- Taxo A bacitracin disk = sensitive

Staphylococcus Species

- G+C content of DNA (moles %) = 30–38
- No teichoic acids in cell wall
- Anaerobic growth and fermentation of glucose
- Anaerobic growth in modified Brewer's
    semisolid thioglycollate medium
- Acid aerobically in glycerol containing 0.4 μg/ml
    of erythromycin
- Sensitive to lysostaphin
- Oxidase (DMSO) negative*
- Colony size on blood agar at 24 hours = 1–3 mm
- Growth at 45°C
- Taxo A bacitracin disk = resistant

*Exception: *Staphylococcus sciuri*

■■■■■■ F I G U R E 4 – 1

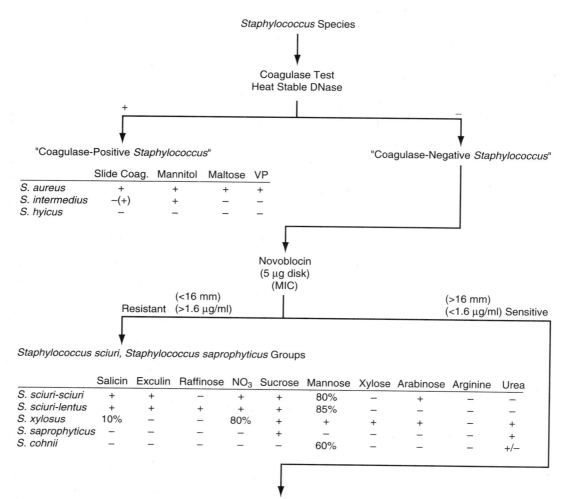

Staphylococcus Species

Coagulase Test
Heat Stable DNase

+

"Coagulase-Positive Staphylococcus"

	Slide Coag.	Mannitol	Maltose	VP
S. aureus	+	+	+	+
S. intermedius	−(+)	+	−	−
S. hyicus	−	−	−	−

−

"Coagulase-Negative Staphylococcus"

Novoblocin
(5 µg disk)
(MIC)

(<16 mm)
Resistant (>1.6 µg/ml)

(>16 mm)
(<1.6 µg/ml) Sensitive

Staphylococcus sciuri, Staphylococcus saprophyticus Groups

	Salicin	Exculin	Raffinose	NO₃	Sucrose	Mannose	Xylose	Arabinose	Arginine	Urea
S. sciuri-sciuri	+	+	−	+	+	80%	−	+	−	−
S. sciuri-lentus	+	+	+	+	+	85%	−	−	−	−
S. xylosus	10%	−	−	80%	+	+	+	+	−	+
S. saprophyticus	−	−	−	−	+	−	−	−	−	+
S. cohnii	−	−	−	−	−	60%	−	−	−	+/−

Staphylococcus Epidermedis, Staphylococcus simulans Groups

	NO₃	Glucose	Sucrose	Mannose	Trehalose	Mannitol	Maltose	Xylose	Lactose	Arginine	Urea
S. epidermidis	86%	+	+	+	−	−	+	−	78%	89%	+
S. hominis	+	+	+	10%	+	7%	+	−	60%	40%	+
S. haemolyticus	+	+	+	−	+	50%	+	−	35%	87%	−
S. warneri	24%	+	+	2%	+	63%	78%	−	11%	25%	−
S. capitis	83%	+	+(s)	+	−	+	−	−	−	76%	87%
S. simulans	+	+	+	78%	78%	+	30%	−	+	+	60%

+ = 90% or greater   % = percentage +
− = 90% or greater   (s) = slow reaction

■■■ F I G U R E 4 - 2

(The reactions and percentages are compiled from strains examined in the Clinical Microbiology Laboratory, University Hospital, The Ohio State University, and from the literature.)

CATALASE

Principle

Members of the staphylococci produce an enzyme, catalase, which reacts with peroxide to liberate oxygen. When a colony is emulsified in 3% hydrogen peroxide, the resultant bubbles on the slide may be visualized, which constitutes a positive test result.

Reagent

3% Hydrogen peroxide

Procedure

1. Place a drop of hydrogen peroxide on a clean glass slide or petri dish.
2. Pick the colony in question from an agar plate with a wooden applicator stick.
3. Touch the stick containing the bacteria to the drop of hydrogen peroxide and observe for immediate bubbling. The reaction is positive if there is a rapid evolution of gas.

Precautions:

The enzyme catalase is present in red cells. Colonies to be tested should not be taken from a blood agar plate directly.

Results

1. Staphylococci are catalase positive.
2. Streptococci are catalase negative.

Quality Control

Controls to verify test performed should be run and recorded daily.

1. *Staphylococcus aureus*—catalase positive
2. *Streptococcus pyogenes*—catalase negative

SLIDE COAGULASE TEST

Principle

Staphylococci produce many extracellular products, but only one is generally accepted as a marker of pathogenic strains: the production of the enzyme coagulase, which clots rabbit and human plasma. Coagulase production is also one of the major criteria used to identify *S. aureus*. All strains of *S. aureus* are, by definition, coagulase positive. There are two kinds of coagulase enzyme: the cell-bound "clumping factor," which is bound to the bacterial cell wall and causes clumping when the bacterial suspension is mixed with plasma, and free coagulase, which is an extracellular enzyme that causes a clot to form when bacterial cells are incubated with the plasma.

This test is used as a screening procedure for organisms having a colonial morphology consistent with *S. aureus*. It detects the production of clumping factor or cell-bound coagulase. Isolates that do not produce bound coagulase must be tested for extracellular free coagulase by the tube test. Therefore, any negative slide coagulase test must be confirmed with the tube coagulase test.

Specimen

A well-isolated colony from a blood agar plate

Reagent

Coagulase plasma: Difco #0286-86-2

Quality Control

1. *S. aureus*—coagulase positive
2. *Staphylococcus epidermidis*—coagulase negative

Procedure continued on following page

Procedure

1. Emulsify a well-isolated colony in a drop of water on a glass slide to produce a dense, uniform suspension. If any evidence of autoagglutination is noted before the plasma is added, the culture is not suitable for the slide test.
2. Add one drop of plasma to the suspension and mix; then rotate 5 seconds.

Results

1. A positive reaction is indicated by easily visible white clumps, which usually appear immediately or within 5 seconds.
2. All negative or questionable results must be confirmed by a tube test.

TUBE COAGULASE TEST

Principle

The tube coagulase test detects the presence of free coagulase enzyme produced by *S. aureus*. This extracellular enzyme forms a clot when bacterial suspension is incubated with the plasma. The screening test by slide method detects only the cell-bound coagulase, and therefore any negative slide coagulase test must be confirmed with the tube coagulase test.

Specimen

A broth culture of the organisms to be tested or a single colony from a blood agar plate

Reagent

Coagulase Plasma: Difco #0286-86-2

Quality Control

1. *S. aureus*—coagulase positive
2. *S. epidermidis*—coagulase negative

Procedure

1. To 0.5 mL of undiluted rabbit plasma, add one loopful of growth from 18- to 24-hour agar culture, 0.1 mL of broth culture, or a single colony from a blood agar plate.
2. Incubate in a water bath at 37°C and examine for clotting at 30-minute intervals for 4 hours.
3. If no clot is observed at the end of 4 hours, let stand at room temperature for 18 to 24 hours. Observe for clotting.

Results

A positive coagulase test result is represented by any degree of clotting from a loose clot suspended in plasma to a solid clot. The majority of coagulase-positive strains produce a clot within 4 hours.

Notes:
1. False-positive test result may occur with mixed cultures or with a pure culture of a gram-negative rod but the clotting mechanism is different.

2. Therefore, organisms to be tested must first be determined to possess characteristics consistent with genus Staphylococcus.

3. S. aureus also produces fibrinolysin enzyme staphylokinase, which lyses the clot. It is important to examine for clot after 4 hours of incubation or a false-negative result may occur.

NOVOBIOCIN SUSCEPTIBILITY TEST

Principle

Staphylococcus saprophyticus is a significant isolate in urine samples of girls. A coagulase-negative staphylococcus (CNS), *S. saprophyticus* must be differentiated from other CNS, such as *S. epidermidis*. *S. saprophyticus* is resistant to 5-μg novobiocin disk, whereas other CNS are susceptible. Other CNS that are resistant to 5-μg novobiocin are *S. xylosus, S. cohni,* and *S. sciuri,* which are uncommon isolates from the urine.

Reagents

5-μg Novobiocin disk (BBL Microbiology Systems, Cockeysville, MD); two sheep blood agar plates

Quality Control

1. *S. epidermidis*—susceptible
2. *S. saprophyticus*—resistant

Procedure

1. Divide a sheep blood agar into two sections and label one half with the positive control and the other with the negative control. Inoculate the control organisms onto their respective sections. Place a 5-μg novobiocin disk at the center of the inoculum. Repeat the procedure using the second sheep blood agar with the test or unknown organism.
2. Incubate the cultures at 35°C in an ambient incubator for 18 to 24 hours. Determine if the test organism is susceptible (equal to or greater than 17 mm) or resistant (less than 17 mm) by measuring the zone of inhibition around the disk.

Results

1. ≥17 mm: susceptible
2. <17 mm: resistant

STREPTOCOCCI

Streptococci are catalase-negative, facultatively anaerobic, gram-positive cocci that usually appear in pairs and chains. Most species are found as normal respiratory tract flora, whereas others are normal flora of the gastrointestinal and urogenital tract. Given the opportunity, these organisms become important agents of human diseases.

Group A β-hemolytic streptococcus, or *Streptococcus pyogenes,* is the most common cause of acute bacterial pharyngitis, scarlet fever, and impetigo. Group B β-hemolytic streptococcus, or *Streptococcus agalactiae,* is the leading cause of meningitis, septicemia, and pneumonia in newborn infants. Group D streptococcus and *Enterococcus* are common isolates from urinary tract and wound infections.

Streptococcus pneumoniae is a common cause of otitis media and purulent sinusitis in young children. Pneumococcal pneumonia with concurrent bacteria often occurs in the elderly and in the presence of predisposing factors, such as alcoholism and chronic obstructive pulmonary disease. *S. pneumoniae* also causes bacterial meningitis in adults.

Viridans streptococci, or α-hemolytic streptococci, inhabit the upper respiratory tract and rarely cause disease. They are the major cause of subacute bacterial endocarditis in patients who have previously damaged heart valve.

The type of hemolysis the organism produces when grown on sheep blood agar is used initially to identify the streptococcus species. There are three types

■■■ T A B L E   4 – 2
PRESUMPTIVE IDENTIFICATION OF STREPTOCOCCI

Test(s)	Group A	Group B	Enterococcus	Group D not Enterococcus	Viridans Non–Group D	Pneumococci
Hemolysis	β	β^*	α, β, γ	α, γ	α, γ	α
Bacitracin	+	$-^*$	–	–	$+^*$	$\pm$
S × T	–	–	–	$+^*$	+	NRL
cAMP	–	+	–	–	–	–
Hippurate	–	+	$-^*$	–	$-^*$	–
Bile-Esculin	–	–	+	+	$-^*$	–
6.5% NaCl	–	$+^*$	+	–	–	–
Optochin and Bile Solubility	–	–	–	–	–	+
Catalase	–	–	–	–	–	–
PYR	+	–	+	–	–	–

* Occasional exceptions occur.
NRL, not recorded in literature.

of hemolysis: α, or incomplete green hemolysis; β, or complete clear hemolysis; and γ, or no hemolysis.

Presumptive identification is made based on the species' susceptibility or resistance to bacitracin (β-hemolytic) or optochin (α-hemolytic) or ability to hydrolyze bile esculin and grow in 6.5% NaCl (nonhemolytic). Definitive identification in some species is made by immunofluorescence or agglutination tests.

Table 4–2 shows the tests that may be used to identify streptococci. Table 4–3 shows the biochemical characteristics of group D streptococcus.

The schema shown in Figure 4–3 describes the presumptive identification of streptococcal species.

Speciation of Group D Streptococcus

Streptococci that are Lancefield type D can be one of six species. These species can be distinguished from each other by a select number of biochemical tests. The names of the species and their biochemical reactions are as follows:

■■■ T A B L E   4 – 3

	bile esculin	6.5% NaCl	Arginine	Lactose	Arabinose	Sorbitol	
Enterococcus faecalis	+	+	+	+	–	+	— Enterococcus
Enterococcus faecium	+	+	+	+	+	–	
Enterococcus durans	+	+	+	+	–	–	
Enterococcus avium	+	+	–	+	+	+	
Streptococcus bovis	+	–	–	+	–	–	— Non-*Enterococcus*
Streptococcus equinus	+	–	–	–	–	–	

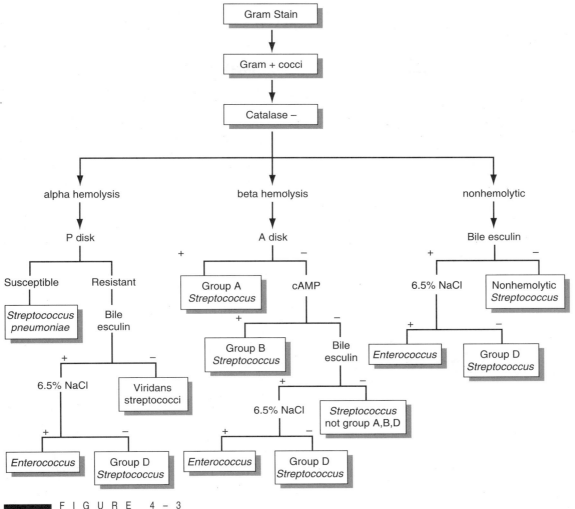

FIGURE 4-3

BACITRACIN INHIBITION TEST USING TAXO A DISK

Principle

To differentiate group A streptococci from other groups of β-hemolytic streptococci, a low concentration of bacitracin selectively inhibits the growth of group A streptococci. A bacitracin disk containing 0.04 units should be used. Accurate determination of hemolysis is crucial because some α-hemolytic streptococci are inhibited by this differential disk. Also, the test is designed for use with a pure culture and not directly on the primary isolation plate. Although rare strains of group A streptococci are bacitracin resistant, approximately 5 to 10% of strains of non–group A β-hemolytic streptococci (primarily group B,C,G) are bacitracin susceptible. Inhibition by bacitracin, therefore, constitutes presumptive identification of group A streptococci.

Reagent

Bacitracin Differential Discs (Taxo A) 0.04 unit Taxo A disks are impregnated with about 0.04 unit of bacitracin per disk. Disks come in a single cartridge of 50 disks. On receipt, store at −20°C. After use, store cartridge to protect integrity at 2 to 8°C. The expiration date applies to product when stored as directed. These disks are for in vitro diagnostic use only.

Quality Control

Check performance weekly with the following control organisms:

- Bacitracin-susceptible group A streptococcus for positive control
- Bacitracin-resistant group B streptococcus for negative control

If results are not acceptable, the procedure should be repeated, using a new cartridge. If results are still not acceptable, retest with a new lot number and discard the reagent. All corrective action taken and the results should be recorded in the "out of control" sheet.

Procedure

1. Transfer isolated colonies to a fresh sheep blood agar plate. Streak the surface of the plate spreading the inoculum into a small area.
2. Aseptically apply a bacitracin disk onto the center of the streaked area.
3. Gently tamp the disk to insure contact with the agar surface.
4. Invert the plate and incubate for 18 hours at 35°C.
5. After incubation, examine the plate for a clear zone of inhibition around the disk.

Results

1. Positive test: any zone of inhibition around the bacitracin disk
2. Negative test: uniform growth right up to the rim of the disk

---

OPTOCHIN SENSITIVITY TEST USING TAXO P DISK

Principle

The optochin sensitivity test is based on the differential susceptibility of S. pneumoniae and other hemolytic streptococci to ethyl hydroxycupreine hydrochloride. S. pneumoniae is inhibited by less than 5 μg/mL of this agent. When contained within a paper disk and applied to an agar surface, as for the disk diffusion antibiotic susceptibility test, the inhibitory zones obtained with S. pneumoniae significantly exceed those obtained with other viridans streptococci.

Reagents

Optochin Disks—Taxo P BBL 31048—Disks are packaged in a single cartridge of 50 disks. Taxo P disks are impregnated with ethyl hydroxycupreine hydrochloride (5.0 μg per disk). On receipt, store at −20°C. After use, store cartridge at 2 to 8°C. Expiration date applies to product when stored as directed. These disks are for in vitro diagnostic use only.

Quality Control

Check performance weekly with the following control organisms:

- S. pneumoniae for positive control
- α-Hemolytic streptococcus (viridans group) for negative control

If results are not acceptable, repeat the procedure using a new cartridge. If the results are still not acceptable, retest using a different lot number and discard old one. All corrective actions taken and the results should be recorded in the "out of control" sheet.

Procedure

1. Streak suspicious colonies on a blood agar plate covering an area 3 cm in diameter.
2. Place an optochin disk in the center of the streaked area, pressing gently with sterile forceps.
3. Invert the plate and incubate at 35 to 37°C for 18 to 24 hours. After incubation, measure the zone of inhibition around the disk.

Expected Results

1. Zone diameter of inhibition   15 mm = S. pneumoniae
2. Zone diameter of inhibition   15 mm = viridans streptococcus group

RAPID HIPPURATE HYDROLYSIS TEST

Principle

Group B β-hemolytic streptococcus produces the enzyme hippuricase, which hydrolyzes sodium hippurate to sodium benzoate and glycine. Subsequent addition of triketohydrindene hydrate (Ninhydrin) results in the oxidative deamination of the α-amino group in glycine. One of the products released is ammonia, which reacts with the residual Ninhydrin to give a purple-colored complex.

Reagents

1. One percent aqueous sodium hippurate solution—dispense 0.4 mL into 13 × 100-mm screw-capped tubes and freeze until used.
2. Ninhydrin reagent

Procedure

1. Remove one tube of hippurate substrate from the freezer for each test and controls and thaw.
2. Inoculate heavily with the bacteria to be tested.
3. Incubate at 37°C for 2 hours.
4. Add approximately 0.2 mL Ninhydrin reagent to each tube.
5. Incubate at 37°C for 10 to 15 minutes.

Results

1. Positive hydrolysis—purple color
2. Negative hydrolysis—colorless

Notes:
Insufficient inoculum may cause weak or false-negative results.

Some strains of enterococci hydrolyze hippurate. These blacken bile-esculin and grow in 6.5% NaCl broth, however.

Some group B streptococci are inhibited by bacitracin disks.

CAMP TEST FOR GROUP B STREPTOCOCCI

Principle

Group B β-hemolytic streptococcus produces an extracellular enzyme, "CAMP" factor (an acronym of the authors who initially described this phenomenon). This CAMP factor intensifies the lysis of sheep red cells when placed in the appropriate inoculation points with *S. aureus*. The β-lysin produced by the staphylococci, in conjunction with the CAMP factor, produces an arrowhead-shaped hemolysis at the junction between the streptococci and staphylococci streaks.

Reagents

5% sheep blood agar (TSA base); *S. aureus* ATCC 25923; group A and group B streptococci control organism

Procedure

1. Inoculate a blood agar plate with *S. aureus* ATCC 25923 by making a single streak across the center of the plate.
2. Streak the test and control organisms at right angles to the Staphylococcus streak, to within 2 mm.
3. Incubate the plate at 35°C overnight or for 5 to 6 hours in a candle jar.
4. Group B streptococci—"arrowhead" of hemolysis.

Note:
Do not incubate the plate anaerobically. Most group A streptococci produce "arrowhead" hemolysis anaerobically.

SALT TOLERANCE TEST

Principle

Enterococci can withstand a higher salt concentration than nonenterococci. A modified broth containing 6.5% NaCl is used. This is used primarily to differentiate enterococci from group D streptococci.

Specimen

Isolated colonies on sheep agar

Medium

Trypticase Soy broth with 6.5% NaCl

Procedure

1. Inoculate one to two colonies into 2 mL of 6.5% NaCl broth.
2. Incubate tube at 35°C for 18 to 24 hours.

Results

1. Positive test: visible turbidity in broth
2. Negative test: no visible turbidity in broth

Note:
The test is inoculum dependent, and too heavy inoculum should be avoided.

BILE ESCULIN TEST

Principle

Group D streptococci can grow in the presence of 40% bile and subsequently hydrolyze esculin. Esculetin, which is the byproduct of esculin hydrolysis, combines with ferric citrate in the medium to give a black complex. The test is used to differentiate group D streptococci and enterococci from other streptococci.

$$\text{Esculin} \xrightarrow{\text{bacterial enzyme}} \text{esculetin} + \text{glucose}$$
$$\text{Esculetin} + Fe^{3+} \rightarrow \text{black complex}$$

Specimen Requirement

Isolated colonies of blood agar

Medium

Bile esculin agar or broth

Procedure

1. Inoculate one to two colonies on a bile esculin agar plate, slant, or broth.
2. Incubate at 35°C for 18 to 24 hours.

Results

1. Positive test: blackening of the agar or of the broth.
2. Negative test: no blackening of the medium. Growth alone does not constitute a positive test.

LABORATORY EXERCISE 1

STAPHYLOCOCCI

Recommended cultures to be studied:

- *S. aureus*
- *S. epidermidis*
- *Micrococcus* sp
- *S. saprophyticus*

Recommended culture media to be used:

- Sheep blood agar
- Phenylethyl alcohol or Columbia CNA
- Chocolate agar
- MacConkey agar

Instructions:

1. Observe and examine the colonial morphology of the following known cultures on each of the inoculated media:

- *S. aureus*
- *S. epidermidis*
- *S. saprophyticus*
- *Micrococcus* sp

2. Prepare smears of each culture and Gram stain.
3. Examine smears.
4. Perform the following biochemical tests:

- Catalase
- Slide coagulase
- Tube coagulase

5. Determine susceptibility of *S. epidermidis* and *S. saprophyticus* to novobiocin disk.
6. Record all results on the laboratory worksheets.

■■■■■■■   LABORATORY WORKSHEET 1

STAPHYLOCOCCI

Student Name _____   Date performed _____
                                                       Date completed _____

Colonial Morphology

Describe the growth and appearance of the organisms.

Culture Medium	Description of Colonies			
	S. aureus	*S. epidermidis*	*Micrococcus* sp	*S. saprophyticus*
Blood agar				
PEA or CNA				
Chocolate agar				
MacConkey agar				

Microscopic Morphology

Describe the cellular morphology of each species. Sketch a
few cells from each smear.

S. aureus

S. epidermidis

Micrococcus sp

S. Saprophyticus

Worksheet continued on opposite page

■■■■■■■ LABORATORY WORKSHEET 1 *Continued*

STAPHYLOCOCCI

Biochemical Reactions
Record Test Results

Tests	Results			
	Micrococcus sp	*S. aureus*	*S. epidermidis*	*S. saprophyticus*
Catalase				
Slide coagulase				
Tube coagulase				

Differentiate *S. epidermidis* from *S. saprophyticus*

Determine if the organism is susceptible or resistant to novobiocin.

Organism	Novobiocin Susceptibility
S. epidermidis	
S. saprophyticus	

■ LABORATORY EXERCISE 2

STREPTOCOCCI

Recommended cultures to be studied:

- Group A β streptococcus (*S. pyogenes*)
- Group B β streptococcus (*S. agalactiae*)
- Enterococcus
- *S. pneumoniae*
- Viridans streptococci

Recommended media to be used:

- Blood agar
- PEA agar
- Chocolate agar
- MacConkey agar

Instructions:

1. Observe and examine the colonial morphology of the above-mentioned organisms. Note each particular type of hemolysis on blood agar.
2. Describe the growth and appearance of these organisms on:
   - Blood agar
   - CNA agar

- Chocolate agar
- MacConkey agar

3. Prepare smears of each culture and Gram stain.
4. Based on the Gram stain, describe the cellular morphology of each species and sketch a few cells from each smear.
5. Perform the following biochemical tests. (PYR test may be used to substitute for A disk susceptibility and 6.5% NaCl tolerance test.)

On β-hemolytic

- A disk
- CAMP
- Bile esculin
- 6.5% NaCl

On α-hemolytic

- "P" disk
- Bile esculin
- 6.5% NaCl

On nonhemolytic

- Bile esculin
- 6.5% NaCl

LABORATORY WORKSHEET 2

Student Name _____

Date performed: _____
Date completed: _____

Colonial Morphology

Describe the growth and appearance of the organisms.

Culture Medium	Description of Colonies				
	Group A Streptococcus	Group B Streptococcus	S. pneumoniae	Enterococcus	Viridans Streptococcus
Blood agar					
PEA/CNA					
Chocolate agar					
MacConkey agar					

Microscopic Morphology

Describe the cellular morphology of each species. Sketch a few cells from each smear.

Group A streptococcus
Gram stain: _____
_____

Group B streptococcus
Gram stain: _____
_____

Worksheet continued on following page

■■■■■■■   LABORATORY WORKSHEET 2 *Continued*

S. pneumoniae

Viridans *streptococcus*

Biochemical Tests

Record results of biochemical tests.

Tests	Results				
	Group A Streptococcus	*Group B Streptococcus*	*S. pneumoniae*	*Enterococcus*	Viridans *Streptococcus*
Catalase					
Bacitracin			✕		✕
CAMP					
Optochin	✕	✕			
Bile esculin					
6.5% NaCl					

CHAPTER 5

Gram-Negative Cocci

This chapter covers *Neisseria* species and *Moraxella catarrhalis,* which are gram-negative cocci.

1. Describe the colonial and microscopic morphology of the members of the genus *Neisseria* and *Moraxella catarrhalis.*

2. Discuss the proper methods of specimen collection and transport for isolation of the significant species.

3. List the appropriate culture media for cultivation.

4. Describe the preliminary and definitive identification schema.

5. Perform the oxidase test and interpret results.

6. Properly inoculate CTA carbohydrates for identification.

7. Given a set of unknown organisms, correctly identify the organism.

NEISSERIA

The genus *Neisseria* consists of oxidase-positive, gram-negative cocci that often appear as kidney bean–shaped diplococci on Gram stain. Most species are normal flora of the mucosa of the respiratory, alimentary, and genital tracts. Certain species such as *Neisseria gonorrhoeae* are recognized as true pathogens. Others such as *Neisseria meningitidis,* which are inhabitants of the oral and upper respiratory flora, may occasionally cause clinical disease. All species grow on blood agar except for *N. gonorrhoeae,* which requires an enriched medium such as chocolate agar or Thayer-Martin agar. Enhanced CO_2 (2 to 8%) is required for optimum incubation atmosphere.

N. gonorrhoeae is a strict pathogen when isolated from any body site. Common sources include the urethra, cervix, and anal canal. Other infections may involve the joints, blood, and conjunctiva. Transport media should be used if the specimen collected is not inoculated immediately to appropriate culture media. Colonies of *N. gonorrhoeae* on Thayer-Martin agar appear small, translucent, grayish, convex, and shiny with entire margins. Suspected colonies are tested for oxidase and a smear is made for Gram stain. Definitive identification is based on carbohydrate utilization or other rapid identification techniques such as latex agglutination.

N. meningitidis is carried as normal nasopharyngeal flora by a large percentage of the population. It is significant, however, when isolated from transtracheal aspirates, cerebrospinal fluid, or blood. In contrast to *N. gonorrhoeae, N. menin-*

gitidis is able to grow on blood agar as well as chocolate agar. The colonies appear small, gray, and convex. Presumptive identification is made based on finding oxidase-positive, gram-negative diplococci. Definitive identification is made by determining utilization of carbohydrates, latex agglutination tests, or fluorescent antibody procedures.

M. catarrhalis is a member of the oral flora that has been recognized as an important agent of lower respiratory infections. Morphologically, these organisms resemble the *Neisseria* species. Definitive identification is based on carbohydrate utilization.

The following chart shows the carbohydrate utilization reactions of *Neisseria* species.

Species	Test/Results CTA Carbohydrates				
	Oxidase	Glucose	Maltose	Lactose	Sucrose
N. gonorrhoeae	+	+	−	−	−
N. meningitidis	+	+	+	−	−
N. lactamica	+	+	+	+	−
M. catarrhalis	+	−	−	−	−

OXIDASE TEST

Principle

Neisseria and some gram-negative rods produce a chemical, indophenol oxidase, which becomes pink to dark red and finally black when colonies come in contact with the oxidase reagent.

Specimen

Isolate colonies growing on blood agar or chocolate plates

Reagent

N_1N_1 Dimethyl-p-phenylenediamine hydrochloride—1.0 g, 2.5 g, 5.0 g; distilled water—100 mL, 250 mL, 500 mL

1. Add the dye to the water and mix with a magnetic stirrer until a faint pink color appears.
2. Fill disposable plastic tubes two-thirds full and place in freezer.

3. When thawed, the reagent is good for 2 to 3 hours.
4. Cepti-Seal Oxidase Reagent is available commercially prepared ready to use.

Procedure

1. Place two to three drops of reagent on a piece of Whatman #1 filter paper.
2. Remove a suspected colony from the plate with a sterile applicator stick and smear onto the reagent saturated paper.

Results

An oxidase-positive reaction is a pink to purple color on the filter paper in 5 to 10 seconds.

GRAM-NEGATIVE COCCI

Instructions: Organisms to be studied:
- *N. gonorrhoeae*
- *N. meningitidis* (if available) or *N. lactamica*
- *M. catarrhalis*

For each culture:

1. Observe the colonies and describe the colonial appearance on the worksheet.
2. Prepare a smear for Gram stain. Stain smear and describe microscopic morphology.
3. Perform an oxidase test and record results on the worksheets.

4. Inoculate a set of Cystine Trypticase Soy Agar (CTA) containing:
   - Glucose
   - Maltose
   - Lactose
   - Sucrose

   Refer to Appendix p. 170 for inoculation procedure for CTA.
5. Incubate all biochemical tests under appropriate atmosphere for 18 to 36 hours. Read and record all results on worksheets.

██████ LABORATORY WORKSHEET

GRAM-NEGATIVE COCCI

Student Name _____

Date performed: _____
Date completed: _____

Colonial Morphology

Describe colonial characteristics.

Culture Medium	Description of Colonies		
Blood agar			
Chocolate agar			
Thayer-Martin			

Microscopic Morphology

Describe microscopic features.

_____   _____

_____   _____

Biochemical Reactions

Species	Tests/Results CTA Carbohydrate Utilization				
	Oxidase	Glucose	Maltose	Lactose	Sucrose

GRAM-POSITIVE AND GRAM-NEGATIVE COCCI

Student Name _____

Date performed: _____
Date completed: _____

Instructions: Given the following cultures taken from:

- ■ Wound
- ■ Throat
- ■ Cerebrospinal fluid

1. Inoculate the appropriate primary media to isolate suspected agents of infectious disease at each of these body sites. Incubate at the proper environmental conditions.

2. After 24 hours of incubation, describe the colonial morphology of each isolate from each culture.
3. Perform all necessary biochemical tests to identify each isolate.
4. Identify all organisms isolated from each culture.

S P E C I M E N: _____

Colonial Morphology: Isolate # _____ BAP Choc Mac Gram Stain:	Biochemical Tests	Identification
Report:		
Colonial Morphology: Isolate # _____ BAP Choc Mac Gram Stain:		
Report:		

Exercise continued on following page

PRACTICE UNKNOWN *Continued*

S P E C I M E N: _____

Colonial Morphology: Isolate # _____ BAP Choc Mac **Gram Stain:**	Biochemical Tests	Identification
Report:		
Colonial Morphology: Isolate # _____ BAP Choc Mac **Gram Stain:**		
Report:		

Exercise continued on opposite page

PRACTICE UNKNOWN *Continued*

S P E C I M E N: _____

Colonial Morphology: Isolate # _____ BAP Choc Mac **Gram Stain:**	Biochemical Tests	Identification
Report:		
Colonial Morphology: Isolate # _____ BAP Choc Mac **Gram Stain:**		
Report:		

·*Exercise continued on following page*

PRACTICE UNKNOWN *Continued*

S P E C I M E N: _____

Colonial Morphology: Isolate # _____
    BAP
    Choc
    Mac
    Gram Stain:
	Biochemical Tests	Identification

Report:		

Colonial Morphology: Isolate # _____
    BAP
    Choc
    Mac
    Gram Stain:		

Report:		

CHAPTER 6

Gram-Positive Bacilli

This section discusses the genera *Corynebacterium* and *Listeria,* which are aerobic, non–spore-forming gram-positive rods.

■■■■■ O B J E C T I V E S

1. Describe the morphology of *Corynebacterium diphtheriae* using Gram stain and Loeffler's methylene blue stain.

2. List the primary isolation media used to cultivate *C. diphtheriae.*

3. Describe the colonial morphology of *C. diphtheriae* on the following media:

   ■ Blood agar

   ■ Loeffler's slants
   ■ Tellurite/Tinsdale

4. Given a set of reactions, differentiate *C. diphtheriae* from other coryneforms.

5. Describe the microscopic and colonial morphology of *Listeria monocytogenes.*

6. Given a set of biochemical reactions, identify and differentiate *Listeria* from other related species.

CORYNEBACTERIUM AND *LISTERIA*

Corynebacteria. The genus *Corynebacterium* is composed of small, gram-positive, pleomorphic rods that may exhibit characteristic palisade or "Chinese letter" arrangements. Some species may tend to have clubbed ends or contain granules that are visible when stained with methylene blue. These granules are sometimes referred to as metachromatic granules or Babès-Ernst bodies. The organisms grow under aerobic conditions, and colonies produced on blood agar are small and usually nonhemolytic. Some strains require special nutrients, such as serum or other animal products, for growth. Selective medium such as Loeffler's agar slant enhances the microscopic morphology of the organism, whereas Tinsdale or tellurite medium inhibits normal oral flora and shows the organism's typical gray or black colonies.

The most clinically significant of these organisms are the toxigenic strains of *C. diphtheriae,* the causative agent of diphtheria. Diphtheria, transmitted by direct contact or by droplet spray, is a respiratory infection that is a localized lesion along the upper respiratory tract. A gray-white membrane is produced from the action of the diphtheria toxin on the epithelium along the site of infection. This membrane may cause fatal complications resulting from mechanical obstruction of the airway. Diphtheria toxin may also be absorbed into the circulation and may cause damage to various organs, particularly the heart.

Because only certain strains of *C. diphtheriae* produce the exotoxin, a virulence test such as the Elek immunodiffusion test is performed.

Other corynebacteria are often referred to as diphtheroids. Diphtheroids are commonly found as members of normal skin flora and other body sites. Other diphtheroids, however, are well-defined species that have been implicated with disease processes, especially among immunodeficient hosts and transplant patients.

Differentiation of *Corynebacterium* sp from other non–spore-forming gram-positive bacilli and other gram-positive organisms is shown in the chart.

Genus and Species	Catalase	Esculin Hydrolysis	Motility	β-Hemolysis	Growth in 6.5% NaCl
Corynebacterium	+	−	−/+	−/+	+/−
L. monocytogenes	+	+	+	+	+
Streptococcus agalactiae	−	−	−	+	−
Enterococci	−	+	−	−/+	+

Listeria. The genus *Listeria* belongs to the family *Listeriaceae,* which includes *L. monocytogenes* and other nonpathogenic *Listeria* spp. *L. monocytogenes* is short, motile, gram-positive non–spore-forming bacillus that occurs in nature, such as soil, vegetation, and water. The organism produces a narrow zone of hemolysis on blood agar, is facultatively anaerobic, produces catalase, and grows over a wide range of temperature on laboratory media. Diagnostic features include a characteristic tumbling motility when observed on hanging drop preparation and an "umbrella" type of growth in semisolid motility medium when incubated at 20 to 25°C.

This organism has been known to cause abortion in sheep and cattle, and cutaneous infections in humans have occurred among veterinarians. Other clinical manifestations include neonatal sepsis and meningitis, sepsis or meningitis among the immunocompromised hosts, and a flu-like illness among pregnant women resulting in infection of the fetus.

Clinical specimens submitted for culture vary depending on the clinical presentation. These sources may include blood, cerebrospinal fluid, amniotic fluid, and, occasionally, genital tract secretions. *L. monocytogenes* grows quite easily on blood agar media and on blood culture media available commercially.

Identification of *L. monocytogenes* is made based on the following biochemical test reactions:

Biochemical Test	Results
Catalase	+
Umbrella motility (25°C)	+
CAMP test	+
Bile esculin	+

Biochemical Test	Results
Acid production Xylose	=
Rhamnose	+
Mannitol	=

Differentiation from other species can be made by demonstrating the characteristic features:

■ Motility at 25°C distinguishes *Listeria* from most *Corynebacterium*.

■ Catalase differentiates them from streptococcus group B (+ CAMP) from *Enterococcus* (+ bile esculin).

A schema for presumptive identification of gram-positive bacilli is given in Figure 6–1.

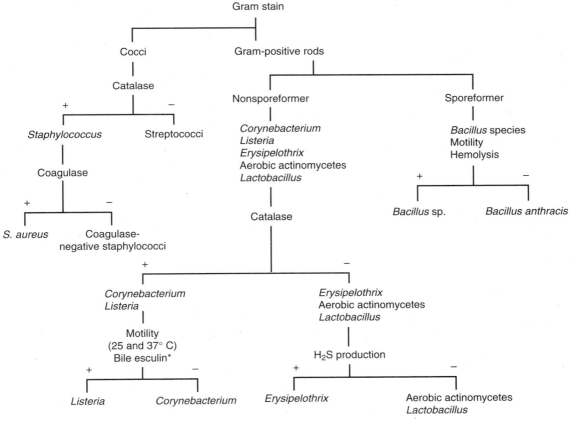

*Except *C. kutcheri*

■■■■■ F I G U R E   6 – 1

(From Larsen H: Gram-positive non–spore-forming rods. In Mahon C, Manuselis G [eds]: Textbook of Diagnostic Microbiology. Philadelphia: WB Saunders, 1995, p. 223.)

MOTILITY TEST IN SEMISOLID AGAR

Principle

The growth of motile organisms in a semisolid medium will be diffused and away from the stab line of inoculation, but that of a nonmotile isolate will be confined to the line of stab. Two agar tubes are used and incubated at 22 to 25°C and 35°C to demonstrate motility of *Listeria* and *Yersinia* at the lower temperature. This test is also used in conjunction with other biochemical tests to identify gram-negative enterics and nonfermenting organisms.

Specimen Requirement

Isolated colony on agar plate

Reagent

Motility test semisolid medium is available commercially prepared. Store at 2 to 8°C; it expires as dated.

Quality Control

1. Positive: *Enterobacter aerogenes*
2. Negative: *Klebsiella pneumoniae*

Controls are run each time the procedure is performed. Quality controls are done each time a new lot is received and monthly thereafter. Record results in the quality control worksheet. If expected results are not obtained, check organism viability and then retest. Record action taken in the "out of control" logsheet.

Procedure

1. Inoculate two motility agar tubes by stabbing halfway down the center of the agar, keeping the inoculating needle as vertical as possible.
2. Leave one tube at room temperature, and incubate the other at 35°C overnight.

Results

Nonmotile bacteria grow only along the line of stab, while the rest of the medium remains clear. Motile bacteria are diffused and away from the stab line, making the medium look hazy to cloudy. *Listeria* grows away from the line of stab, and an umbrella-like pattern of growth can be seen several millimeters below the agar surface, giving the medium a cloudy appearance. Greater motility of *Listeria* is observed with agar incubated at room temperature than at 35°C.

Spore-Formers

This section covers the aerobic or facultatively anaerobic, gram-positive spore-forming rods of *Bacillus*.

OBJECTIVES

1. Describe the colonial and microscopic morphology of *Bacillus* species.

2. Based on microscopic morphology, differentiate spore-forming gram-positive bacilli from other gram-positive rods.

3. Given the microscopic morphology and growth requirements, identify an unknown organism to the genus level.

BACILLUS

The genus *Bacillus* includes several species that are facultatively anaerobic, gram-positive bacilli that produce endospores. Most strains are saprophytic and traditionally have been clinically insignificant. Several reports have been published implicating certain *Bacillus* species in serious infections predominantly among immunosuppressed individuals.

Bacillus anthracis is the primary human pathogen in this genus and the causative agent of anthrax. Infections may result from handling animal hides or wool from infected animals such as sheep and cattle. Clinical manifestations may be cutaneous, pulmonary, or gastrointestinal, depending on the route of transmission. Inhaling the spores results in the pulmonary form (woolsorter's disease), and entrance of the organism through open cuts and abrasions manifests as a cutaneous lesion (malignant pustule). Indirect transmission occurs by ingestion of uncooked contaminated meat or unpasteurized contaminated milk.

B. anthracis is a large, nonmotile, square-ended, facultative anaerobe that produces centrally located endospores. The cells, which frequently occur in chains, give a "bamboo" appearance when seen microscopically. On blood agar, the colonies are nonhemolytic and usually are large, raised, and irregular. Strict safety precautions are mandatory when working with cultures of *B. anthracis*.

Bacillus cereus is another facultatively anaerobic gram-positive bacillus that is recognized as a cause of food poisoning. The two distinct clinical manifestations include diarrhea, which is associated with contaminated meat and sauces, and vomiting, which results from eating contaminated rice dishes. Laboratory diagnosis of food poisoning due to *B. cereus* includes quantitative cultures of food samples. Isolation of the organism from stool is not diagnostic because *B. cereus* can be found in normal stool.

■■■■ ■■■■ LABORATORY EXERCISE 1

CORYNEBACTERIUM/LISTERIA

Recommended cultures to be studied:

- *Corynebacterium* sp
- *L. monocytogenes*
- Group B streptococcus (*S. agalactiae*)

Recommended culture media to be used:

- Sheep blood agar
- Loeffler serum agar slant (*Corynebacterium*)
- Tinsdale or tellurite (*Corynebacterium*)

Instructions:

1. Observe the colonial morphology of *Corynebacterium* sp on blood agar and compare the morphology with the colonies of other gram-positive non–spore-forming rods.
2. Describe the morphology of *Corynebacterium* sp on Loeffler's serum agar slant and tellurite media. Describe the morphology of *L. monocytogenes* and compare with group B streptococci.
3. Prepare smears of each organism for Gram stain from the blood agar isolates. Prepare another of *Corynebacterium* sp from the Loeffler's agar slants for methylene blue stain.
4. Stain and examine the smears. Describe the cellular morphology. Sketch a few cells from each smear.
5. Perform a catalase test on each organism.
6. Inoculate the following biochemical test media with *L. monocytogenes* and group B streptococci:
   - Motility test at 25 to 35°C
   - CAMP test
   - Bile esculin
7. Incubate for 18 to 24 hours.
8. Record all results on the worksheets provided.

██████████ LABORATORY WORKSHEET

CORYNEBACTERIUM/LISTERIA

Student Name _____

Date performed: _____
Date completed: _____

Colony Morphology

Describe the growth and appearance of the colonies on each medium.

Culture Medium	Description of Colonies		
	L. monocytogenes	S. agalactiae	Corynebacterium
Blood agar plate			

Microscopic Morphology

Describe the microscopic morphology of each organism examined.

Gram stain

S. agalactiae

Corynebacterium

L. monocytogenes

Corynebacterium sp
Gram stain
_____

Corynebacterium sp
Loeffler's methylene blue
_____

Worksheet continued on following page

████████ LABORATORY WORKSHEET *Continued*

Biochemical Tests

Biochemical Tests	Results		
	L. monocytogenes	*S. agalactiae*	*Corynebacterium*
Catalase			
Motility 25/35°C			
Bile esculin			
CAMP			

BACILLUS

Instructions: Recommended organisms to be studied are *B. cereus* and *Bacillus subtilis*.

Note: B. anthracis is a highly infectious bacterial agent. Therefore, laboratory exercises are performed using stock cultures of saprophytic species such as *B. cereus* and *B. subtilis*.

Colony Morphology

1. Observe the growth of the above-mentioned stock cultures on blood agar.

2. Describe the colonial morphology.

Microscopic Morphology

1. Prepare a smear for Gram stain.
2. Observe and describe the characteristic microscopic morphology.
3. Sketch a few cells on the space provided.

█████████   LABORATORY WORKSHEET

BACILLUS

Student Name _____

Date performed: _____
Date completed: _____

Colony Morphology

Culture	Description of Colonies	
	B. cereus	*B. subtilis*
Blood agar plate		

Microscopic Morphology

B. cereus
Gram stain: _____

B. subtilis
Gram stain: _____

CHAPTER 7

Enterobacteriaceae

This chapter covers the most commonly encountered members of the family *Enterobacteriaceae:* those that cause opportunistic infections and those that are true intestinal pathogens.

■■■■■ O B J E C T I V E S

1. List the general characteristics of the family *Enterobacteriaceae.*

2. Inoculate and interpret results from the following biochemical tests:

   ■ TSI agar slant
   ■ LIA agar slant
   ■ Oxidase test
   ■ Urease
   ■ Voges-Proskauer
   ■ SIM

   ■ Citrate
   ■ Nitrate reduction
   ■ Methyl red test

3. Explain the principle for each of the above-mentioned test reactions.

4. Given a set of results, be able to identify an unknown organism.

5. List additional tests needed for complete identification.

6. Inoculate and interpret results of the API 20E or any miniaturized identification system.

GENERAL CHARACTERISTICS

The family *Enterobacteriaceae* is composed of gram-negative bacilli that inhabit the large intestine of humans and animals and thereby have been referred to as enteric bacilli. These organisms are also ubiquitous in soil, water, and decaying matter. Except for the true intestinal pathogens that cause typhoid fever and bacillary dysentery, most enteric bacilli do not cause disease. Given the opportunity to invade other body sites outside their habitat, however, these organisms are able to produce severe infections. Most common hospital-acquired infections, such as urinary tract infections, respiratory infections, and wound infections, are caused by this group of organisms.

Clinical specimens submitted for isolation of enterics include sputum, body fluids, pus, tissues, rectal swabs, and feces. When rectal swabs and fecal specimens are received in the laboratory, intestinal pathogens are suspected.

Morphology

The members of the family *Enterobacteriaceae* are small, gram-negative, non–spore-forming rods and are facultatively anaerobic. They may possess a well-defined capsule and pili may be present in most species. Lipopolysaccharide (LPS) is a major component of the cell wall responsible for the endotoxic effects produced during enteric infections. When grown on nonselective media such as blood agar, chocolate agar, and brain heart infusion agar, enterics produce large, gray, smooth colonies. Highly selective and differential media are frequently used for isolation and presumptive identification of intestinal significant pathogens.

Antigenic Properties

The antigenic structures—capsule (K), cell wall (O), and flagella (H)—are significant in the identification and epidemiologic studies of this group of organisms. Capsular antigens (K) are heat-labile polysaccharides that can mask the heat-stable somatic (O) antigens. In some species, such as *Salmonella typhi,* this capsular antigen functions as a virulence factor.

Somatic (O) cell wall antigen is the LPS component of the cell wall. This heat-stable antigen is useful as a serologic marker. It is most significant, however, because it also serves as a virulence factor that causes the toxic effects of enteric infections.

Flagellar (H) antigens are proteins. These antigens are particularly helpful in the classification and serologic speciation of members of the genus *Salmonella.*

Biochemical Characteristics

Enterics are biochemically diverse. By definition, all members ferment glucose, reduce nitrate to nitrites, and are oxidase negative. They may be motile or nonmotile and may or may not produce gas. Fermentation of glucose by most species is by the mixed acid pathway, whereas others use the butanediol fermentative pathway, which is a useful distinguishing characteristic between genera. These reactions are described fully in Chapter 16, *Textbook of Diagnostic Microbiology.*

Lactose Fermentation

The reaction patterns shown here are an integral part of the family *Enterobacteriaceae* identification schema. Composition of KIA and TSI agar and the principle of the reactions produced are described in the Appendix, pp 181 and 216.

Reactions on KIA or TSI agar:

1. Nonfermenter: alkaline slant/alkaline deep (ALK/ALK) or (ALK/NC)

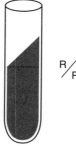

R/R

2. Nonlactose fermenter: acid slant/acid deep (8 to 12 hours)

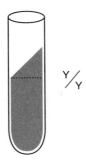

3. Alkaline slant/acid deep (Alk/Acid) (18 to 24 hours)

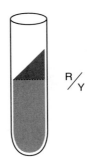

4. Alkaline/acid (black deep) H_2S produced

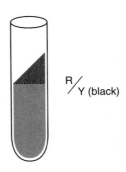

5. Lactose (sucrose) fermenter: acid/acid

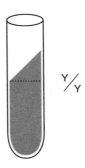

OPPORTUNISTIC *ENTEROBACTERIACEAE*

Escherichia coli

Escherichia coli inhabits the large intestine of humans and is the most common facultative gram-negative isolate from the colon flora. This species is the number one cause of urinary tract infections. It is also known to cause neonatal meningitis; traveler's diarrhea; and other opportunistic infections, such as pneumonia, wounds, and bacteremia.

E. coli ferments lactose rapidly. It produces large, usually β-hemolytic, gray colonies on blood agar. On MacConkey agar, colonies appear dry, flat, and dark pink in color owing to the fermentation of lactose present in the medium. The following are typical biochemical reactions for presumptive identification:

■■■■■■■■ IMViC FORMULA (INDOLE, METHYL RED, VOGES-PROSKAUER, CITRATE)

Indole	+ positive
Methyl red	+ positive
Voges-Proskauer	− negative
Citrate	− negative

Klebsiella, Enterobacter, Serratia, and *Hafnia*

These species are commonly found in the gastrointestinal tract or free living in nature. They are usually associated with nosocomial infections, particularly pneumonia, urinary tract, and wound infections. These organisms are biochemially similar, and presumptive identification of an oranism belonging to this group can be made if it exhibits the following IMViC formula:

Indole   −
Methyl Red   −
Voges-Proskauer   +
Citrate   +

These reactions, however, may be variable for any given species, and therefore additional confirmatory tests must be performed before final identification is made. Representative species are discussed subsequently.

Klebsiella pneumoniae (Friedlander's bacillus) is the major cause of classic lobar pneumonia among hospitalized patients. Clinical manifestations include abscess formation and necrosis. Distinctive features seen in the laboratory include the absence of motility and the presence of polysaccharide capsule, which is responsible for the mucoid appearance of the colonies.

Enterobacter species are common opportunistic pathogens found in nosocomial and mixed infections. Some strains have been isolated from contaminated intravenous fluids. Species are differentiated from *Klebsiella* by motility and except for *Enterobacter agglomerans* the ability to decarboxylate ornithine.

Serratia species are also opportunistic pathogens that are commonly associated with nosocomial infections. They are found in nature, particularly in soil, water, plants, and animals. They ferment lactose slowly, with some strains taking 3 to 4 days. Members of this genus are differentiated from other enterobacteria by the ability to produce extacellular DNase. Species identification is based on fermentation of carbohydrates and decarboxylase activity. *Serratia rubidaea* and *Serratia marcescens* both form red pigments. *Serratia liquefaciens* is the third species of this genus that causes human infections.

Proteus, Providencia, and Morganella

The feature of this group that distinguishes it from other *Enterobacteriaceae* is its ability to deaminate phenylalanine. These organisms are normally found in soil, water, and sewage and in the intestinal tract of humans. Clinical infections include urinary tract and wound infections as well as pneumonia and septicemia.

Proteus mirabilis and *Proteus vulgaris* both have the ability to swarm over the surface of an enriched medium, producing a thin sheet of growth. Neither species ferments lactose, but both produce hydrogen sulfide and urease. Differentiation between the two species is made based on the ability of *P. vulgaris* to produce indol.

Morganella morganii and *Providencia rettgeri* are two species that were formerly classified under the genus *Proteus*. Using DNA homology studies, it was found that both are less closely related to *Proteus*. Both species produce urease, but neither produces hydrogen sulfide nor swarms.

Morganella morganii and *Providencia* species are often associated with nosocomial infections involving the urinary tract, respiratory tract, and wounds.

Edwardsiella tarda is the only species in the tribe. The organism has been isolated from wounds, blood, and spinal fluids and from feces from patients with gastroenteritis. *E. tarda* does not ferment lactose and produces hydrogen sulfide, which may cause this organism to be confused with *Salmonella*. *E. tarda,* however, produces indole.

Figure 7–1 is a schematic diagram for the presumptive identification of commonly encountered *Enterobacteriaceae*. Additional biochemical tests must be performed for definitive identification and confirmation.

INTESTINAL PATHOGENS: *SALMONELLA, SHIGELLA,* AND *YERSINIA*

Salmonella

Salmonella causes a wide variety of infections in animals and humans. Human infections may include extraintestinal invasion of tissues and enteric fevers. *Salmonella* species possess antigenic structures that are used for serologic grouping. The O and H antigens are the major antigens used to type the

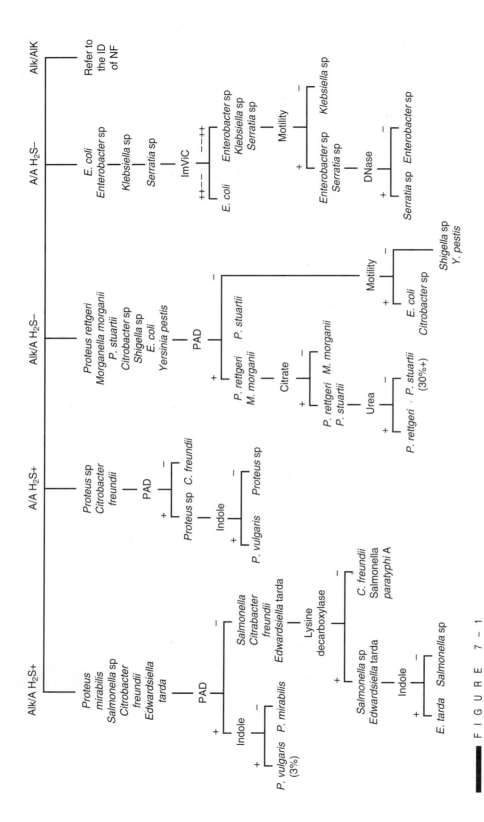

F I G U R E 7 - 1

IMViC: indole, methyl-red, Voges-Proskauer, citrate; PAD: phenylalanine deaminase; Alk/A: alkaline/acid; A/A: acid/acid; H₂S⁺: hydrogen sulfide positive; H₂S⁻: hydrogen sulfide negative; NF: nonfermenter; g: gas.

KOVAC'S INDOLE TEST

Principle

This test is used primarily to differentiate the members of the family *Enterobacteriaceae* and other miscellaneous gram-negative bacteria. The production of red color indicates indole has been produced from the amino acid tryptophan.

Specimen

48-hour culture of organisms in broth that contains tryptophan

Reagent

■ Amyl or isoamyl alcohol, 150 mL
■ p-Dimethylaminobenzaldehyde, 10 g
■ Hydrochloric acid, conc., 50 mL

Dissolve aldehyde in alcohol and then slowly add acid. The dry aldehyde should be light in color. Alcohols that result in

indole reagents that become deep brown in color should not be used.

Quality Control

1. *E. coli:* indole positive
2. *K. pneumoniae:* indole negative

Procedure

1. Add about 0.5 mL of Kovac's reagent to 24- to 48-hour culture incubated at 37°C and shake the tube gently.
2. A deep red color develops in the presence of indole.
3. Test may be done at 24 hours, but if this is done, 1 or 2 mL of culture should be removed aseptically for testing.
4. If test result is negative, the remaining culture should be reincubated for an additional 24 hours.

NITRATE REDUCTION TEST

Principle

Nitrate reduction test is used for identification of gram-negative bacilli. Reduction of nitrate is indicated by the development of a red color within a few minutes after reagents are added to the culture medium. However, no color development may indicate either nitrate is not reduced or nitrate is reduced beyond nitrite to ammonia or nitrogen.

Specimen Requirement

24- to 48-hour culture of the organism in nitrate broth

Reagents

1. Solution A

■ Sulfanilic acid, 2 g, 8 g
■ Acetic acid (5N), 250 mL, 1000 mL
2. Solution B
■ α-Naphthylamine, 1.2 g, 5g
■ Acetic acid (5N), 250 mL, 1000 mL

To make 5N acetic acid:
■ Glacial acetic acid, 200 mL, 400 mL
■ Distilled water, 500 mL, 1000 mL

Procedure

1. Inoculate the nitrate broth medium with test organism and incubate for 24 to 48 hours.
2. Test for nitrate reduction by adding five drops of each solution A and solution B. Shake gently.
3. Let stand for 1 to 2 minutes.

Results

1. A red color develops if the test is positive for nitrate reduction.
2. No color production is a negative test result and should be confirmed by the addition of zinc dust. If unreduced nitrate is present, a red color develops confirming the negative test. If no color change occurs, a complete reduction has occurred, and the test result is positive.

species. The numerous antigenic types of the genus are arranged in such a way that the members are grouped into major groups, designated by capital letters A through I based on common O antigens.

The groups are subdivided into serotypes by determining the remaining O antigens and H antigens. There are approximately 2000 serotypes of *Salmonella;* however, only 38% of the serotypes account for 95% of all clinical isolates. The capsular antigen Vi (virulence) of *Salmonella typhi* plays an important role as a determinant of pathogenicity. In the laboratory diagnosis of *S. typhi,* the Vi antigen may prevent the detection of the presence of O antigen.

Salmonella does not ferment lactose (with rare exceptions), is motile, and produces H$_2$S and gas from glucose fermentation. Differentiation from members of other genera is shown in Table 7–1.

Shigella

Bacillary dysentery is caused by organisms that belong to the genus *Shigella,* which are strict pathogens and are only found in humans. They rarely cause disease in animals. Infections most often occur among the younger population, particularly in children and infants in developing countries.

There are four species in the genus *Shigella: S. dysenteriae, S. flexneri, S. boydii,* and *S. sonnei.* Speciation is based on biochemical reactions and serogrouping.

Shigella species are divided into four major groups depending on their O antigens: group A, B, C, D, which corresponds to *S. dysenteriae, S. flexneri, S. boydii, S. sonnei.* Some species may possess K antigens that may block the O antigen during serologic grouping. This interference can be eliminated by boiling the bacterial suspension to remove the heat-labile capsular antigen. Because all *Shigella* are nonmotile, they do not possess flagellar (H) antigens.

Other biochemical characteristics include no fermentation of lactose, no production of hydrogen sulfide, and no production of gas from glucose except for some species of S. flexneri. Because these organisms are closely related to *Escherichia, Shigella* may be differentiated from *Escherichia* by its inability to use acetate as a source of carbon and inability to decarboxylate lysine.

Yersinia

Members of the genus *Yersinia* are primarily animal pathogens. Humans occasionally acquire infections through direct or indirect contact. The organisms are gram-negative coccobacilli that show bipolar staining, sometimes described as a "safety pin appearance." These organisms belong to the family *Enterobacteriaceae* because their metabolic and growth requirements are similar to those of enteric organisms. The genus includes organisms that cause diarrheal diseases and also includes the agent that causes plague, *Y. pestis.*

Yersinia enterocolitica has been recognized as an important cause of gastroenteritis in humans, characterized by fever, diarrhea, and abdominal pain. Enterocolitis caused by this organism is attributed to its invasiveness and to an endotoxin it produces. It may also cause mesenteric lymphadenitis, in which symptoms may mimic that of acute appendicitis. Isolation of this organism requires cold enrichment.

Laboratory diagnosis of *Salmonella, Shigella,* and *Yersinia* infections includes the isolation of the organisms from feces. Blood cultures are appropriate for the detection of septicemia in patients suspected of having typhoid fever or other enteric fevers.

■■■■■■ T A B L E   7 – 1

BIOCHEMICAL REACTIONS OF THE NAMED SPECIES, BIOGROUPS, AND ENTERIC GROUPS OF THE FAMILY ENTEROBACTERIACEAE*

Species	Indole Production	Methyl Red	Voges-Proskauer	Citrate (Simmons)	Hydrogen Sulfide (TSI)	Urea Hydrolysis	Phenylalanine Deaminase	Lysine Decarboxylase	Arginine Dihydrolase	Ornithine Decarboxylase	Motility (36°C)	Gelatin Hydrolysis (22°C)	Growth in KCN	Malonate Utilization	D-Glucose, Acid	D-Glucose, Gas	Lactose Fermentation	Sucrose Fermentation	D-Mannitol Fermentation	Dulcitol Fermentation
Buttiauxella																				
B. agrestis	0	100	0	100	0	0	0	0	0	100	100	0	80	60	100	100	100	0	100	0
Cedecea																				
C. davisae†	0	100	50	95	0	0	0	0	50	95	95	0	86	91	100	70	19	100	100	0
C. lapagei†	0	40	80	99	0	0	0	0	80	0	80	0	100	99	100	100	60	0	100	0
C. neteri†	0	100	50	100	0	0	0	0	100	0	100	0	65	100	100	100	35	100	100	0
Cedecea sp. 3†	0	100	50	100	0	0	0	0	100	0	100	0	100	0	100	100	0	50	100	0
Cedecea sp. 5†	0	100	50	100	0	0	0	0	50	50	100	0	100	0	100	100	0	100	100	0
Citrobacter																				
C. freundii†	5	100	0	95	80	70	0	0	65	20	95	0	96	15	100	95	50	30	99	55
C. diversus†	99	100	0	99	0	75	0	0	65	99	95	0	0	90	100	98	35	45	100	50
C. amalonaticus†	100	100	0	85	0	80	0	0	85	95	98	0	95	0	100	97	50	15	100	0
C. amalonaticus biogroup 1†	100	100	0	1	0	45	0	0	85	100	99	0	96	0	100	93	19*	100	100	4
Edwardsiella																				
E. tarda†	99	100	0	1	100	0	0	100	0	100	98	0	0	0	100	100	0	0	0	0
E. tarda biogroup 1†	100	100	0	0	0	0	0	100	0	100	100	0	0	0	100	50	0	100	100	0
E. hoshinae	13	100	0	0	0	0	0	100	0	95	100	0	0	100	100	35	0	100	100	0
E. ictaluri	0	0	0	0	0	0	0	100	0	65	0	0	0	0	100	50	0	0	0	0
Enterobacter																				
E. aerogenes†	0	5	98	95	0	2	0	98	0	98	97	0	98	95	100	100	95	100	100	5
E. cloacae†	0	5	100	100	0	65	0	0	97	96	95	0	98	75	100	100	93	97	100	15
E. agglomerans†	20	50	70	50	0	20	20	0	0	0	85	2	35	65	100	20	40	75	100	15
E. gergoviae†	0	5	100	99	0	93	0	90	0	100	90	0	0	96	100	98	55	98	99	0
E. sakazakii†	11	5	100	99	0	1	50	0	99	91	96	0	99	18	100	98	99	100	100	0
E. taylorae†	0	5	100	100	0	1	0	0	94	99	99	0	98	100	100	100	10	0	100	0
E. amnigenus biogroup 1†	0	7	100	70	0	0	0	0	9	55	92	0	100	91	100	100	70	100	100	0
E. amnigenus biogroup 2†	0	65	100	100	0	0	0	0	35	100	100	0	100	100	100	100	35	0	100	0
E. intermedium	0	100	100	65	0	0	0	0	0	89	89	0	65	100	100	100	100	65	100	100
Escherichia-Shigella																				
E. coli†	98	99	0	1	1	1	0	90	17	65	95	0	3	0	100	95	95	50	98	60
E. coli, inactive†	80	95	0	1	1	1	0	40	3	20	5	0	1	0	100	5	25	15	93	40
Shigella, serogroups A, B, and C†	50	100	0	0	0	0	0	0	5	1	1	0	0	0	100	2	0	0	93	2
S. sonnei†	0	100	0	0	0	0	0	0	2	98	0	0	0	0	100	0	2	1	99	0
E. fergusonii†	98	100	0	17	0	0	0	95	5	100	93	0	0	35	100	95	0	0	98	60
E. hermanii†	99	100	0	1	0	0	0	6	0	100	99	0	94	0	100	97	45	45	100	19
E. vulneris†	0	100	0	0	0	0	0	85	30	0	100	0	15	85	100	97	15	8	100	0
E. blattae	0	100	0	50	0	0	0	100	0	100	0	0	0	100	100	100	0	0	0	0
Ewingella																				
E. americana†	0	84	95	95	0	0	0	0	0	0	60	0	5	0	100	0	70	0	100	0
Hafnia																				
H. alvei†	0	40	85	10	0	4	0	100	6	98	85	0	95	50	100	98	5	10	99	0
H. alvei biogroup 1	0	85	70	0	0	0	0	100	0	45	0	0	0	45	100	0	0	0	55	0
Klebsiella																				
K. pneumoniae†	0	10	98	98	0	95	0	98	0	0	0	0	98	93	100	97	98	99	99	30
K. oxytoca†	99	20	95	95	0	90	1	99	0	0	0	0	97	98	100	97	100	100	99	55
Klebsiella group 47 indole positive, ornithine positive†	100	96	70	100	0	100	0	100	0	100	0	0	100	100	100	100	100	100	100	10
K. planticola†	20	100	98	100	0	98	0	100	0	0	0	0	100	100	100	100	100	100	100	15
K. ozaenae†	0	98	0	30	0	10	0	40	6	3	0	0	88	3	100	50	30	20	100	2
K. rhinoscleromatis†	0	100	0	0	0	0	0	0	0	0	0	0	80	95	100	0	75	100	100	0
K. terrigena	0	60	100	40	0	0	0	100	0	20	0	0	100	100	100	80	100	100	100	20
Kluyvera																				
K. ascorbata†	92	100	0	96	0	0	0	97	0	100	98	0	92	96	100	93	98	98	100	25
K. cryocrescens†	90	100	0	80	0	0	0	23	0	100	90	0	86	86	100	95	95	81	95	0
Moellerella																				
M. wisconsensis	0	100	0	80	0	0	0	0	0	0	0	0	70	0	100	0	100	100	60	0
Morganella																				
M. morganii†	98	97	0	0	5	98	95	0	0	98	95	0	98	1	100	90	1	0	0	0
M. morganii biogroup 1†	100	95	0	0	41	100	100	100	0	95	0	0	91	5	100	91	0	0	0	0
Obesumbacterium																				
O. proteus biogroup 2	0	15	0	0	0	0	0	100	0	100	0	0	0	0	100	0	0	0	0	0

Salicia Fermentation	Adonitol Fermentation	myc-Inositol Fermentation	D-Sorbitol Fermentation	L-Arabinose Fermentation	Raffinose Fermentation	L-Rhamnose Fermentation	Maltose Fermentation	D-Xylose Fermentation	Trehalose Fermentation	Cellubiose Fermentation	α-Methyl-D-Glucoside Fermentation	Erythritol Fermentation	Esculin Hydrolysis	Melibiose Fermentation	D-Arabitol Fermentation	Glycerol Fermentation	Mucate Fermentation	Tartrate, Jordan	Acetate Utilization	Lipase (Corn Oil)	DNase at 25°C	Nitrite → Nitrate	Oxidase, Kovacs	ONPG‡	Yellow Pigment	D-Mannose Fermentation
100	0	0	0	100	100	100	100	100	100	100	0	0	100	100	0	60	100	60	0	0	0	100	0	100	0	100
99	0	0	0	0	10	0	100	100	100	100	5	0	45	0	100	0	0	0	0	91	0	100	0	90	0	100
100	0	0	0	0	0	0	100	0	100	100	0	0	100	0	100	0	0	0	60	100	0	100	0	100	0	100
100	0	0	100	0	0	0	100	100	100	100	0	0	100	0	100	0	0	0	0	100	0	100	0	100	0	100
100	0	0	0	0	100	0	100	100	100	100	50	0	100	100	100	0	0	0	50	100	0	100	0	100	0	100
100	0	0	100	0	100	0	100	100	100	100	0	0	100	100	100	0	0	0	50	50	0	100	0	100	0	100
5	0	3	98	100	30	99	99	99	99	55	5	0	0	50	0	98	95	90	80	0	0	99	0	95	0	100
20	98	0	99	100	0	100	100	100	100	99	40	0	2	0	100	98	93	75	75	0	0	100	0	96	0	100
40	0	0	100	100	5	99	99	99	100	100	5	0	10	5	0	70	98	85	75	0	0	99	0	100	0	100
0	0	0	100	100	100	100	100	100	100	100	70	0	0	0	0	55	100	93	82	0	0	100	0	100	0	100
0	0	0	0	9	0	0	100	0	0	0	0	0	0	0	0	30	0	25	0	0	0	100	0	0	0	100
0	0	0	0	100	0	0	100	0	0	0	0	0	0	0	0	0	0	0	0	0	0	100	0	0	0	100
50	0	0	0	13	0	0	100	0	100	0	0	0	0	0	0	65	0	0	0	0	0	100	0	0	0	100
0	0	0	0	0	0	0	100	0	0	0	0	0	0	0	0	0	0	0	0	0	0	100	0	0	0	100
100	98	95	100	100	96	99	99	100	100	100	95	0	98	99	100	98	90	95	50	0	0	100	0	100	0	95
75	25	15	95	100	97	92	100	99	100	99	85	0	30	90	15	40	75	30	75	0	0	99	0	99	0	100
65	7	15	30	95	30	85	89	93	97	55	7	0	60	50	30	30	40	25	30	0	0	85	0	90	75	98
99	0	0	0	99	97	99	100	99	100	99	2	0	97	97	97	100	2	97	93	0	0	99	0	97	0	100
99	0	75	0	100	99	100	100	100	100	100	96	0	100	100	0	15	1	1	96	0	0	99	0	100	98	100
92	0	0	1	100	0	100	99	100	100	100	1	0	90	0	0	1	75	0	35	0	0	100	0	100	0	100
91	0	0	9	100	100	100	100	100	100	100	55	0	91	100	0	0	35	9	0	0	0	100	0	91	0	100
100	0	0	100	100	0	100	100	100	100	100	100	0	100	100	0	100	0	0	0	0	0	100	0	100	0	100
100	0	0	100	100	100	100	100	100	100	100	100	0	100	100	0	100	100	100	0	0	0	100	0	100	0	100
40	5	1	94	99	50	80	95	95	98	2	0	0	35	75	5	75	95	95	90	0	0	100	0	95	0	98
10	3	1	75	85	15	65	80	70	90	2	0	0	5	40	5	65	30	85	40	0	0	98	0	45	0	97
0	0	0	30	60	50	5	30	2	80	0	0	0	0	50	0	10	0	30	2	0	0	100	0	2	0	100
0	0	0	2	95	3	75	90	2	100	5	0	0	0	25	0	15	10	90	0	0	0	100	0	90	0	100
65	98	0	0	98	0	92	96	96	96	96	0	0	46	0	100	20	0	96	0	0	0	100	0	83	0	100
40	0	0	0	100	40	97	100	100	100	97	0	0	40	0	8	3	97	35	78	0	0	98	0	98	98	100
30	0	0	1	100	99	93	100	100	100	100	25	0	20	100	0	25	78	2	30	0	0	100	0	100	50	100
0	0	0	0	100	0	100	100	100	75	0	0	0	0	0	0	100	50	50	0	0	0	100	0	0	0	100
80	0	0	0	0	0	23	16	13	99	10	0	0	50	0	99	24	0	35	10	0	0	97	0	85	0	99
13	0	0	0	95	2	97	100	98	99	15	0	0	7	0	0	95	0	70	15	0	0	100	0	90	0	100
55	0	0	0	0	0	0	0	0	70	0	0	0	0	0	0	0	0	30	0	0	0	100	0	30	0	100
99	90	95	99	99	99	99	98	99	99	98	90	0	99	99	98	97	90	95	75	0	0	99	0	99	0	99
100	99	98	99	98	100	100	100	100	100	100	98	2	100	99	98	99	93	98	90	0	0	100	0	100	1	100
100	100	95	100	100	100	100	100	100	100	100	100	0	100	100	100	100	96	100	95	0	0	100	0	100	0	100
100	100	100	92	100	100	100	100	100	100	100	100	0	100	100	100	100	100	100	62	0	0	100	0	100	1	100
97	97	55	65	98	98	90	55	95	95	98	92	70	0	80	97	95	65	25	50	2	0	80	0	80	0	100
98	100	95	100	100	90	96	100	100	100	100	0	0	30	100	100	50	0	50	0	0	0	100	0	0	0	100
100	100	80	100	100	100	100	100	100	100	100	100	0	100	100	100	100	100	20	0	0	0	100	0	100	0	100
100	0	0	40	100	98	100	100	99	100	100	98	0	99	99	0	40	90	35	50	0	0	100	0	100	0	100
100	0	0	45	100	100	100	100	91	100	100	95	0	100	100	0	5	81	19	86	0	0	100	0	100	0	100
0	100	0	0	0	100	0	30	0	0	0	0	0	100	75	10	0	30	10	0	0	0	90	0	90	0	100
0	0	0	0	0	0	0	0	0	10	0	0	0	0	0	0	5	0	95	0	0	0	90	0	5	0	98
0	0	0	0	0	0	0	0	0	0	0	0	0	0	0	0	100	0	100	0	0	0	91	0	0	0	95
0	0	0	0	0	0	15	50	15	85	0	0	0	0	0	0	0	0	15	0	0	0	100	0	0	0	85

Table continued on following page

━━━ T A B L E   7 – 1

BIOCHEMICAL REACTIONS OF THE NAMED SPECIES, BIOGROUPS, AND ENTERIC GROUPS OF THE FAMILY ENTEROBACTERIACEAE* *Continued*

Species	Indole Production	Methyl Red	Voges-Proskauer	Citrate (Simmons)	Hydrogen Sulfide (TSI)	Urea Hydrolysis	Phenylalanine Deaminase	Lysine Decarboxylase	Arginine Dihydrolase	Ornithine Decarboxylase	Motility (36°C)	Gelatin Hydrolysis (22°C)	Growth in KCN	Malonate Utilization	D-Glucose, Acid	D-Glucose, Gas	Lactose Fermentation	Sucrose Fermentation	D-Mannitol Fermentation	Dulcitol Fermentation
Proteus																				
P. mirabilis†	2	97	50	65	98	98	98	0	0	99	95	90	98	2	100	96	2	15	0	0
P. vulgaris†	98	95	0	15	95	95	99	0	0	0	95	91	99	0	100	85	2	97	0	0
P. penneri†	0	100	0	0	30	100	99	0	0	0	85	50	99	0	100	45	1	100	0	0
P. myxofaciens	0	100	100	50	0	100	100	0	0	0	100	100	100	0	100	100	0	100	0	0
Providencia																				
P. rettgeri†	99	93	0	95	0	98	98	0	0	0	94	0	97	0	100	10	5	15	100	0
P. stuartii†	98	100	0	93	0	30	95	0	0	0	85	0	100	0	100	0	2	50	10	0
P. alcalifaciens†	99	99	0	98	0	0	98	0	0	1	96	0	100	0	100	85	0	15	2	0
P. rustigianii†	98	65	0	15	0	0	100	0	0	0	30	0	100	0	100	35	0	35	0	0
Rahnella																				
R. aquatilis†	0	88	100	94	0	0	95	0	0	0	6	0	0	100	100	98	100	100	100	88
Salmonella																				
Subgroup 1 serotypes†—most	1	100	0	95	95	1	0	98	70	97	95	0	0	0	100	96	1	1	100	96
S. typhi†	0	100	0	0	97	0	0	98	3	0	97	0	0	0	100	0	1	0	100	0
S. choleraesuis†	0	100	0	25	50	0	0	95	55	100	95	0	0	0	100	95	0	0	98	5
S. paratyphi A†	0	100	0	0	10	0	0	0	15	95	95	0	0	0	100	99	0	0	100	90
S. gallinarum†	0	100	0	0	100	0	0	90	10	1	0	0	0	0	100	0	0	0	100	90
S. pullorum†	0	90	0	0	90	0	0	100	10	95	0	0	0	0	100	90	0	0	100	0
Subgroup s strains†	2	100	0	100	100	0	0	100	90	100	98	2	0	95	100	100	1	1	100	90
Subgroup 3a strains† (Arizona)	1	100	0	99	99	0	0	99	70	99	99	0	1	95	100	99	15	1	100	0
Subgroup 3b strains† (Arizona)	2	100	0	98	99	0	0	99	70	99	99	0	1	95	100	99	85	5	100	1
Subgroup 4 strains†	0	100	0	98	100	2	0	100	70	100	98	0	95	0	100	100	0	0	98	0
Subgroup 5 strains†	0	100	0	100	100	0	0	100	100	100	100	0	100	0	100	80	0	0	100	100
Serratia																				
S. marcescens†	1	20	98	98	0	15	0	99	0	99	97	90	95	3	100	55	2	99	99	0
S. marcescens biogroup 1†	0	100	60	30	0	0	0	55	4	65	17	30	70	0	100	0	4	100	96	0
S. liquefaciens group†	1	93	93	90	0	3	0	95	0	95	95	90	90	2	100	75	10	98	100	0
S. rubidaea†	0	20	100	95	0	2	0	55	0	0	85	90	25	94	100	30	100	99	100	0
S. odorifera biogroup 1†	60	100	50	100	0	5	0	100	0	100	100	95	60	0	100	0	70	100	100	0
S. odorifera biogroup 2†	50	60	100	97	0	0	0	94	0	0	100	94	19	0	100	13	97	0	97	0
S. plymuthica†	0	94	80	75	0	0	0	0	0	0	50	60	30	0	100	40	80	100	100	0
S. ficaria†	0	75	75	100	0	0	0	0	0	0	100	100	55	0	100	0	15	100	100	0
"Serratia" fonticola†	0	100	9	91	0	13	0	100	0	97	911	0	70	88	100	79	97	21	100	91
Tatumella																				
T. ptyseos†	0	0	5	2	0	0	90	0	0	0	0	0	0	0	100	0	0	98	0	0
Yersinia																				
Y. enterocolitica†	50	97	2	0	0	75	0	0	0	95	2	0	2	0	100	5	5	95	98	0
Y. frederiksenii†	100	100	0	15	0	70	0	0	0	95	5	0	0	0	100	40	40	100	100	0
Y. intermedia†	100	100	5	5	0	80	0	0	0	100	5	0	10	5	100	18	35	100	100	0
Y. kristensenii†	30	92	0	0	0	77	0	0	0	92	5	0	0	0	100	23	8	0	100	0
Y. pestis†	0	80	0	0	0	5	0	0	0	0	0	0	0	0	100	0	0	0	97	0
Y. pseudotuberculosis†	0	100	0	0	0	95	0	0	0	0	0	0	0	0	100	0	0	0	100	0
"Yersinia" ruckeri	0	97	10	0	0	0	0	50	5	100	0	30	15	0	100	5	0	0	100	0
Xenorhabdus																				
X. luminescens (25°C)	50	0	0	50	0	25	0	0	0	0	100	50	0	0	75	0	0	0	0	0
X. nematophilus (25°C)	40	0	0	0	0	0	0	0	0	0	100	80	0	0	80	0	0	0	0	0
Enteric group 17†	0	100	2	100	0	60	0	0	21	95	0	0	97	3	100	95	75	100	100	0
Enteric group 41†	100	100	0	0	0	50	0	0	0	0	100	0	100	50	100	100	100	100	100	100
Enteric group 45†	0	100	0	100	0	0	0	100	22	100	100	0	78	0	100	89	0	0	100	0
Enteric group 57†	0	70	0	40	100	0	0	0	0	0	0	0	30	0	100	60	0	0	0	50
Enteric group 58†	0	100	0	85	0	70	0	100	0	85	100	0	100	85	100	85	30	0	100	85
Enteric group 59†	10	100	0	100	0	0	30	0	60	0	100	0	80	90	100	100	80	0	100	0
Enteric group 60†	0	100	0	0	0	50	0	0	0	100	75	0	0	100	100	0	0	0	50	0
Enteric group 63	0	100	0	0	0	0	0	100	0	100	65	0	0	100	100	0	0	0	100	0
Enteric group 64	0	100	0	50	0	0	0	0	50	0	100	0	100	100	100	50	100	0	100	0
Enteric group 68†	0	100	50	0	0	0	0	0	0	0	0	0	100	0	100	0	0	100	100	0
Enteric group 69	0	0	100	100	0	0	0	0	100	100	100	0	100	100	100	100	100	25	100	100

* Each number gives the percentage of positive reactions after 2 days' incubation at 36°C (except *Xenorhabdus*, which was incubated at 25°C). The vast majority of these positive reactions occur within 24 hrs. Reactions that become positive after 2 days are not considered.

† Known to occur in clinical specimens.

‡ ONPG, *o*-nitrophenyl-β-galactopyranoside.

From Farmer JJ II, Davis BR, Hickman-Brenner FW, et al: Biochemical identification of new species and biogroups of Enterobacteriaceae isolated from clinical specimens. J Clin Microbiol 21:46, 1985. Reprinted by permission.

Salicin Fermentation	Adonitol Fermentation	myo-Inositol Fermentation	D-Sorbitol Fermentation	L-Arabinose Fermentation	Raffinose Fermentation	L-Rhamnose Fermentation	Maltose Fermentation	D-Xylose Fermentation	Trehalose Fermentation	Cellobiose Fermentation	α-Methyl-D-Glucoside Fermentation	Erythritol Fermentation	Esculin Hydrolysis	Melibiose Fermentation	D-Arabitol Fermentation	Glycerol Fermentation	Mucate Fermentation	Tartrate, Jordan	Acetate Utilization	Lipase (Corn Oil)	DNase at 25°C	Nitrate → Nitrite	Oxidase, Kovacs	ONPG‡	Yellow Pigment	D-Mannose Fermentation
0	0	0	0	0	1	1	0	98	98	1	0	0	0	0	0	70	0	87	20	92	50	95	0	0	0	0
50	0	0	0	0	1	5	97	95	30	0	60	1	50	0	0	60	0	80	25	80	80	98	0	1	0	0
0	0	0	0	0	1	0	100	100	55	0	80	0	0	0	0	55	0	85	5	45	40	90	0	1	0	0
0	0	0	0	0	0	0	100	0	100	0	100	0	0	0	0	100	0	100	0	100	50	100	0	0	0	0
50	100	90	1	0	5	70	2	10	0	3	2	75	35	5	100	60	0	95	60	0	0	100	0	5	0	100
2	5	95	1	1	7	1	0	1	7	98	5	0	0	0	0	0	50	0	90	75	0	10	100	0	10	0	100
1	98	1	1	1	1	0	1	1	2	1	0	0	0	0	0	0	15	0	90	40	0	0	100	0	1	0	100
0	0	0	0	0	0	0	0	0	0	0	0	0	0	0	0	0	5	0	50	25	0	0	100	0	0	0	100
100	0	0	94	100	94	94	94	94	100	100	0	0	100	100	0	13	30	6	6	0	0	100	0	100	0	100
0	0	35	95	99	2	95	97	97	99	5	2	0	5	95	0	5	90	90	90	0	2	100	0	2	0	100
0	0	0	99	2	0	0	97	82	100	0	0	0	0	100	0	20	0	100	0	0	0	100	0	0	0	100
0	0	0	90	0	1	100	95	98	0	0	0	1	0	45	1	0	0	85	1	0	0	98	0	0	0	95
0	0	0	95	100	0	100	95	0	100	5	0	0	0	95	0	10	0	0	0	0	0	100	0	0	0	100
0	0	0	1	80	10	10	90	70	50	10	0	1	0	0	0	0	50	100	0	0	10	100	0	0	0	100
0	0	0	10	100	1	100	5	90	90	5	0	0	0	0	0	0	0	0	0	0	0	100	0	0	0	100
5	0	5	100	100	0	100	100	100	100	0	8	0	15	8	0	25	96	50	95	0	0	100	0	15	0	95
0	0	0	99	99	1	99	98	100	99	1	1	0	1	95	1	10	90	5	90	0	2	100	0	100	0	100
0	0	0	99	99	1	99	98	100	99	1	1	0	1	95	1	10	20	75	2	0	2	100	0	100	0	100
60	5	0	100	100	0	98	100	100	100	50	0	0	0	100	5	0	0	65	70	0	0	100	0	100	0	100
0	0	0	100	100	0	100	100	100	100	0	0	0	0	75	0	0	100	0	100	0	0	100	0	100	0	100
95	40	75	99	0	2	0	96	7	99	5	0	1	95	0	0	95	0	75	50	98	98	98	0	95	0	99
92	30	30	92	0	0	0	70	0	100	4	0	0	96	0	0	92	0	50	4	75	82	83	0	75	0	100
97	5	60	95	98	85	15	98	100	100	5	5	0	97	75	0	95	0	75	40	85	85	100	0	93	0	100
99	99	20	1	100	99	1	99	99	100	94	1	0	94	99	85	20	0	70	80	99	99	100	0	100	0	100
98	50	100	100	100	100	95	100	100	100	100	0	0	95	100	0	40	5	100	60	35	100	100	0	100	0	100
45	55	100	100	100	7	94	100	100	100	0	7	0	40	96	0	50	0	100	65	65	100	100	0	100	0	100
94	0	50	65	100	94	0	94	94	100	88	70	0	81	93	0	50	0	100	55	70	100	100	0	70	0	100
100	0	55	100	100	70	35	100	100	100	8	0	100	40	100	0	0	17	40	77	100	92	8	100	0	100
100	100	30	100	100	100	76	97	85	100	6	91	0	100	98	100	88	0	58	15	0	0	100	0	100	0	100
55	0	0	0	0	11	0	0	9	93	0	0	0	0	25	0	7	0	0	0	0	0	98	0	0	0	100
20	0	30	99	98	5	1	75	70	98	75	0	0	25	1	40	90	0	85	15	55	5	98	0	95	0	100
92	0	20	100	100	30	99	100	100	100	100	0	0	85	0	0	85	5	55	15	55	0	100	0	100	0	100
100	0	15	100	100	45	100	100	100	100	0	96	77	100	80	45	60	6	88	18	12	0	94	0	90	0	100
15	0	15	10	77	0	0	100	85	100	100	0	0	0	0	45	70	0	40	8	0	0	100	0	70	0	100
70	0	0	50	100	0	1	80	90	100	0	0	0	50	20	0	50	0	0	0	0	0	85	0	50	0	100
25	0	0	0	50	15	70	95	100	100	0	0	0	95	70	0	50	0	50	0	0	0	95	0	70	0	100
0	0	0	50	5	5	0	95	0	95	5	0	0	0	0	0	50	0	30	0	30	0	75	0	50	0	100
0	0	0	0	0	0	0	25	0	0	0	0	0	0	0	0	0	0	50	0	0	0	0	0	0	50	100
0	0	0	0	0	0	0	0	0	0	0	0	0	0	0	0	0	0	60	0	0	20	20	0	0	60	80
100	0	0	100	100	70	5	100	97	100	100	95	0	95	0	0	11	21	30	87	0	0	100	0	100	0	100
100	100	0	0	100	100	100	100	100	100	100	0	0	100	100	100	0	100	100	0	0	0	100	0	100	100	100
11	0	0	0	100	22	100	100	100	100	100	0	0	55	80	0	0	0	13	55	0	0	89	0	80	0	100
0	0	0	0	90	0	0	0	90	0	0	0	0	0	0	0	60	0	0	0	0	0	0	0	0	0	0
100	0	0	100	100	0	100	100	100	100	100	55	0	0	0	0	30	0	60	45	0	0	100	0	100	0	100
100	0	0	0	100	0	100	100	100	100	100	10	0	100	0	0	10	60	50	50	0	0	100	0	100	25	100
0	0	0	0	25	0	75	0	0	100	0	0	0	0	0	0	75	0	75	0	0	0	100	0	100	0	100
100	0	0	100	100	0	100	100	100	100	100	65	0	100	0	0	0	65	0	0	0	0	100	0	100	0	100
100	100	0	0	100	0	100	100	100	100	100	0	0	100	0	100	0	100	50	0	0	0	100	0	100	0	100
50	0	0	0	0	0	0	50	0	100	0	0	0	0	0	0	50	0	0	0	0	100	0	0	0	0	100
100	0	0	100	100	100	100	100	100	100	100	100	0	100	100	0	0	100	0	25	0	0	100	0	100	100	100

■■■■■■■ LABORATORY EXERCISE 1

OPPORTUNISTIC *ENTEROBACTERIACEAE*

Recommended cultures to be studied:
- *E. coli*
- *E. aerogenes*
- *P. mirabilis*
- *S. marcescens*
- *K. pneumoniae*
- *P. vulgaris*
- *Citrobacter freundii*
- *E. tarda*

Recommended culture media to be inoculated to study colonial morphology and growth characteristics:
- Blood agar
- MacConkey
- Hektoen enteric (HE)
- XLD

These organisms are selected because each species demonstrates either the positive or negative reaction for each of the tests to be performed.

Instructions:

1. Observe and examine the colonial morphology of the following organisms on blood agar, MacConkey, HE, and XLD.

2. Prepare smears of each culture from the blood agar and stain with Gram stain.
3. Examine each smear and describe microscopic morphology. Sketch a few cells.
4. Do an oxidase test on each organism.
5. Inoculate the following (recommended) biochemical tests with each organism. Refer to the Appendix for inoculation procedure and interpretation of results as indicated.
   - TSI agar slant (Appendix p. 216)
   - Simmons Citrate (Appendix p. 166)
   - Urea (Appendix p. 220)
   - LIA (Appendix p. 185)
   - MR/VP (Appendix p. 191)
   - Nitrate reduction
   - Indole Test
   - Motility or SIM
6. Incubate the cultures for 18 to 24 hours at 35 to 37°C.
7. Read and record all results on worksheets provided.

███████ LABORATORY WORKSHEET

Colony Morphology

Organism	Blood Agar	MacConkey Agar

Worksheet continued on following page

■■■■■■   LABORATORY WORKSHEET *Continued*

Biochemical Test Reactions

Tests	E. coli	K. pneumoniae	E. aerogenes	P. vulgaris
TSI				
Nitrate reduction				
Indole/motility				
Citrate				
Urea				
MR/VP				
LIA				
Oxidase				

OTHER ORGANISMS TESTED

Tests				
TSI				
Nitrate reduction				
Indole/motility				
Citrate				
Urea				
MR/VP				
LIA				
Oxidase				

■■■■■■ LABORATORY EXERCISE 2

INTESTINAL PATHOGENS: *SALMONELLA, SHIGELLA, YERSINIA*

Instructions:

1. Observe and examine the colony morphology of *Salmonella, Shigella,* and *P. vulgaris* species on blood agar, MacConkey, HE, and XLD.
2. Inoculate the following biochemical test media with each organism:
   - TSI agar
   - Urea
   - LIA

   - Indole
   - Citrate
   - Motility or SIM
3. Incubate all cultures at 37°C for 18 to 24 hours.
4. Read and record all results.
5. Perform serologic identification using the following antisera:
   - *Salmonella* species: group A, B, C_1, C_2, D, E, Vi; polyvalent antisera
   - *Shigella* species: group A, B, C, D; alkalescens-dispar

██████ LABORATORY WORKSHEET

SALMONELLA, SHIGELLA, PROTEUS VULGARIS

Student Name _____

Date performed: _____
Date completed: _____

Colony Morphology

Organism	Culture Media			
	BAP	MAC	HE	XLD
Salmonella enteritidis				
Shigella sp				
P. vulgaris				

Biochemical Test Reactions

Organism	Tests/Results				
	TSI	Indole/Motility	Citrate	Urea	LIA
S. enteritidis					
Shigella sp					
P. vulgaris					

Organisms	*Salmonella* Antisera Group							
	A	B	C1	C2	D	E	V1	Poly
Positive control								
Negative control								
Unknown								

CHAPTER 8

Vibrio, Aeromonas, *and* Campylobacter

This chapter covers other agents of diarrheal diseases and infections caused by species of *Vibrio, Aeromonas,* and *Campylobacter.*

■■■■■ O B J E C T I V E S

1. Describe the microscopic morphology of organisms that belong to the genera *Vibrio, Aeromonas,* and *Campylobacter.*

2. List the special nutrient and selective media to isolate these organisms.

3. Describe the colonial morphology of these organisms on these selective media.

4. List the biochemical tests used to presumptively identify these groups of organisms.

5. Name the confirmatory tests commonly used to identify these organisms.

VIBRIO

The vibrios belong to the family *Vibrionaceae,* which includes three clinically significant genera: *Vibrio, Aeromonas,* and *Pleisomonas.*

Vibrio species are curved gram-negative rods that may occasionally join together forming S shapes. These organisms live primarily in water and are found naturally in marine animals. They most often cause intestinal diseases; however, they have also been isolated from extraintestinal sites, such as wounds and ears, that have come in contact with seawater. Most infections result from ingestion of insufficiently cooked seafood or contaminated drink and water injuries. There are several important species in this genus: *Vibrio cholerae,* the causative agent of cholera; *V. parahaemolyticus, V. alginolyticus,* and *V. vulnificus.* Refer to the *Textbook of Diagnostic Microbiology* for a complete discussion of *V. cholerae.*

Vibrio species that are not *V. cholerae* are sometimes referred to as "halophilic vibrios." *V. parahaemolyticus, V. alginolyticus,* and *V. vulnificus* are in this group. *V. parahaemolyticus* causes intestinal illness whose clinical manifestations include cramping, watery diarrhea, abdominal pains, and low-grade fever. It usually results from ingestion of insufficiently cooked seafood. *V. alginolyticus* has been associated with infections of cuts and wounds contaminated with seawater. *V. vulnificus* produces clinical infections, such as necrotizing wounds and primary septicemia, that become metastatic lesions. Most patients involved are those with underlying diseases, especially liver disorders.

Specimens submitted for culture are feces and rectal swabs, although the organisms have been isolated from blood and wound cultures. Halophilic vibrios require a high concentration of salt for cultivation, and therefore special selective media are required for isolation of these organisms. Thiosulfate citrate bile sucrose (TCBS) agar is used along with an alkaline peptone broth supplemented with 3% NaCl.

Biochemical differentiation of the important species of the family *Vibrionaceae* is shown in the following table:

Species	Growth in NaCl				VP	Lysine	Lactose	Sucrose
	0%	3%	6%	8%				
V. alginolyticus	−	+	+	+	+	+	+	+
V. cholerae	+	+	+/−	−	+/−	+	−	+
V. parahaemolyticus	−	+	+	+	−	+	−	−
V. vulnificus	−	+	+	−	−	+	+	−

VP, Voges-Proskauer

AEROMONAS

The members of the genus *Aeromonas* are free-living organisms found in water. Most species except for one, *Aeromonas hydrophila,* do not cause human disease. *A. hydrophila* has been known to cause clinical infections such as septicemia, wounds, abscesses, and diarrheal illness. These organisms grow readily on ordinary media; however, they are often misidentified as an enteric, both morphologically and biochemically. The oxidase test is positive for *Aeromonas* spp, which excludes this organism from the family *Enterobacteriaceae.* Usual specimens submitted for culture are feces and rectal swabs, although the organisms have been isolated from blood and wound cultures.

The genus *Pleisomonas,* although uncommon, has also been isolated from blood and spinal fluid but primarily from feces. The following table shows the differentiating characteristics between *Vibrio* and *Aeromonas:*

Characteristics	*Vibrio*	*Aeromonas*
Na⁺ requirement for growth	+	−
Oxidase	+	+
Sensitivity to 0129 vibriostatic compound	+	−
Polar flagella	+	−

CAMPYLOBACTER

A new agent of diarrheal disease in humans, *Campylobacter jejuni,* has been recognized as a cause of abortions in sheep and cattle. Since 1973, this agent has been associated with infectious diarrhea characterized by clinical features such as fever, abdominal pains, and bloody watery stools.

Campylobacter spp are curved gram-negative rods. These organisms are oxidase positive and microaerophilic and require 42°C for growth. They also require a selective medium, made of brucella agar, sheep blood, and a combination of antimicrobials: vancomycin, bacitracin, cephalothin, amphotericin B, trimethroprim, polymyxin B. Skirrow and CAMPY-BAP are examples of this type of medium.

The following table shows the diagnostic features for identification of *Campylobacter* species:

Species	Growth at			Susceptible to Nalidixic Acid	Cephalothin	Hippurate Hydrolysis
	25°C	*37°C*	*42°C*			
C. jejuni	−	+	+	S	R	+
C. fetus	+	+	−	R	S	−
C. coli	−	+	+	S	R	−

■■■■■■■   LABORATORY EXERCISE 1

VIBRIO, AEROMONAS, AND CAMPYLOBACTER

Instructions: Recommended organisms to be studied:

■ *Vibrio parahaemolyticus*
■ *Vibrio alginolyticus*
■ *Aeromonas hydrophila*
■ *Campylobacter jejuni*

Campylobacter

1. Observe and examine the colonial morphology of *C. jejuni* on CAMPY agar medium.
2. Perform the following procedures:
   ■ Prepare a smear and Gram stain. Observe the microscopic morphology.
   ■ Perform an oxidase and catalase test.
   ■ Subculture the organism to 3 BAP and incubate at 25, 35, and 42°C.
   ■ Perform a susceptibility test using nalidixic acid and cephalothin antimicrobial disks.
3. Read and record all results.

Aeromonas

1. Observe the colonial morphology of *A. hydrophila* on blood agar, MacConkey.

2. Perform the following procedures:
   ■ Prepare a smear and Gram stain. Describe the microscopic morphology and record results.
   ■ Do an oxidase test.
   ■ Inoculate the following biochemicals—TSI and API 20E—and incubate all cultures at 37°C for 18 to 24 hours.
3. Read and record all results.

Vibrio

1. Observe the colonial morphology of *V. parahaemolyticus,* *V. alginolyticus,* and *Aeromonas* sp on blood agar, MacConkey, and TCBS.
2. Perform the following procedures:
   ■ Prepare a smear from the colony and Gram stain. Describe the microscopic morphology and record results.
   ■ Perform catalase and oxidase tests.
   ■ Inoculate the following biochemical test media—TSI, VP, lysine, lactose, sucrose, Nutrient broth with NaCl (0%, 3%, 6%, 8%)—and incubate all cultures for 18 to 24 hours at 37°C.
3. Read and record all results.

██████████ LABORATORY WORKSHEET

CAMPYLOBACTER

Student Name _____

Date performed: _____
Date completed: _____

Colony Morphology

Colony Morphology	CAMPY BAP
Campylobacter jejuni	

Microscopic Morphology

Campylobacter

Biochemical Tests

Tests	*Campylobacter jejuni* Test Results
Oxidase	
Catalase	
Growth at 25°C _____	
35°C _____	
42°C _____	
Nalidixic acid susceptibility	
Cephalothin susceptibility	

LABORATORY WORKSHEET

VIBRIO

Colony Morphology

Species	Description of Colonies		
	BAP	MacConkey	TCBS
V. parahaemolyticus			
V. alginolyticus			
Aeromonas sp			

Microscopic Morphology

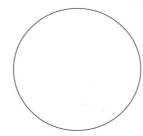
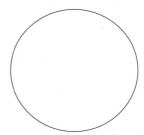

V. parahaemolyticus   V. alginolyticus   Aeromonas sp

Biochemical Test Results

Tests	V. parahaemolyticus	V. alginolyticus	Aeromonas sp
Oxidase			
Catalase			
TSI			
VP			
Lysine			
Lactose			
Sucrose			
Nutrient broth with NaCl			
0%			
3%			
6%			
8%			

■■■■■■ LABORATORY EXERCISE 2

INTESTINAL PATHOGENS

Student Name _____

Date performed: _____
Date completed: _____

Instructions: Given the following stool cultures:
1. Describe the colonial morphology of each isolate from each culture.
2. Perform appropriate biochemical tests to identify the organisms isolated.

3. Record all tests performed and results in the worksheets provided.
4. Give the identification of the organisms isolated.

■■■■■■ S P E C I M E N: _____

Colonial Morphology: Isolate # _____
   BAP
   Choc
   Mac
   HE
   XLD
 Gram Stain:
	Biochemical Tests	Identification

Report:		

Colonial Morphology: Isolate # _____
   BAP
   Choc
   Mac
   HE
   XLD
 Gram Stain:		

Report:		

Exercise continued on following page

LABORATORY EXERCISE 2 *Continued*

S P E C I M E N: _____

Colonial Morphology: Isolate # _____	Biochemical Tests	Identification
BAP Choc Mac HE XLD **Gram Stain:**		
Report:		
Colonial Morphology: Isolate # _____ BAP Choc Mac HE XLD **Gram Stain:**		
Report:		

Exercise continued on opposite page

■■■■■ S P E C I M E N: _____

Colonial Morphology: Isolate # _____ BAP Choc Mac HE XLD **Gram Stain:**	Biochemical Tests	Identification
Report:		
Colonial Morphology: Isolate # _____ BAP Choc Mac HE XLD **Gram Stain:**		
Report:		

Exercise continued on following page

LABORATORY EXERCISE 2 *Continued*

S P E C I M E N: _____

Colonial Morphology: Isolate # _____
   BAP
   Choc
   Mac
   HE
   XLD
Gram Stain:
	Biochemical Tests	Identification

Report:		

Colonial Morphology: Isolate # _____
   BAP
   Choc
   Mac
   HE
   XLD
Gram Stain:		

Report:		

CHAPTER 9

Pseudomonas and Other Nonfermenting Gram-Negative Rods

This chapter discusses the genus *Pseudomonas* and other opportunistic nonfermenting gram-negative rods such as *Acinetobacter* and *Moraxella*.

■ OBJECTIVES

1. Describe distinguishing colonial morphology of *Pseudomonas aeruginosa*.

2. List the biochemical tests used to presumptively identify *Pseudomonas* species and *Acinetobacter* species.

3. Differentiate nonfermenting organisms from fermenting gram-negative rods.

4. Describe the differences between *Pseudomonas, Acinetobacter,* and *Moraxella* species.

PSEUDOMONAS

Members of the genus *Pseudomonas* are ubiquitous in nature. They are found free living most especially in moist environments. Except for *P. aeruginosa,* most species are superficial colonizers and are frequently isolated as contaminants. These organisms, however, have gained significance as infectious agents among immunocompromised hosts.

P. aeruginosa is a nonfermenting organism often associated with opportunistic infections, including urinary tract, respiratory, bacteremia, and infections of severe burns. It is an aerobic, motile, gram-negative rod and produces water-soluble pigment pyocyanin and a fluorochrome pigment pyoverdin, causing green coloration on the culture medium. This species does not require special nutrient for growth and grows over a wide range of temperature and environment.

MORAXELLA

The genus *Moraxella* consists of gram-negative coccobacilli that may appear in pairs. This morphologic characteristic along with a positive oxidase reaction has caused the misidentification and confusion of this organism with the genus *Neisseria*. *Moraxella* species, particularly *Moraxella lacunata,* have been occasionally associated with conjunctival infections.

ACINETOBACTER

The genus *Acinetobacter* consists of organisms that are gram-negative coccobacilli that do not ferment carbohydrates. They are found in nature and have been considered as colonizers and contaminants. Isolation of these organisms from clinical specimens, however, warrants further investigation of the patient's clinical history because they have been associated with significant infections among immunosuppressed hosts.

The two species of clinical importance are *Acinetobacter calcoaceticus* var *iwoffi* and *Acinetobacter baumanii*. Both organisms are common agents of nosocomial respiratory and urinary tract infections.

PROCEDURE FOR OXIDATION-FERMENTATION (O-F) TEST

Principle

This test is used to demonstrate whether the bacteria use carbohydrates fermentatively or oxidatively. In fermentation, pyruvic acid ultimately transfers its electrons to organic compounds with the formation of a large amount of mixed acids. In oxidation, pyruvic acid further enters the Krebs cycle, where it ultimately transfers its electrons to oxygen to form water. Citric acid produced in the Krebs cycle is a weak acid compared with the mixed acids produced by fermentation. O-F medium is specifically formulated to detect weak acidity because it contains a lower amount of peptone, the metabolism of which yields less alkaline amine to neutralize any acid that has been produced, and a high carbohydrate content.

Glucose or another carbohydrate is added to a final concentration of 1% and brom thymol blue is incorporated as an indicator. Two tubes of O-F glucose are inoculated, one of which is overlaid with sterile mineral oil to create an anaerobic environment (for fermentation) and the other of which is exposed to atmospheric oxygen (for oxidation).

Specimen

Growth on agar slant or plate

Reagent

O-F glucose 1% is available commercially prepared. Store at 2 to 8°C. O-F glucose expires as dated.

Quality Control

■ Glucose oxidizer: *P. aeruginosa*
■ Glucose nonoxidizer: *Alcaligenes faecalis*
■ Glucose fermenter: *Klebsiella pneumoniae*

Controls are run each time the procedure is performed. Quality controls are done each time a new lot number is received and monthly thereafter. Record all results in the quality control worksheet. If expected results are not obtained, test for organism viability and retest. Record all actions taken in the "out of control" logsheet.

Procedure

1. Inoculate bacterial growth from the slant or a plate into two tubes of O-F glucose medium. *Note:* If O-F medium has been in the refrigerator, bring it to a boil for 5 minutes to let the air out. Let cool before inoculating.
2. Overlay one tube (closed) with five drops of sterile mineral oil. Do not add mineral oil to the second tube.
3. Incubate at 35°C for 18 to 24 hours.

Results

The medium remains blue if no acid is formed and becomes yellow when acid is formed. There are three possible reactions:

1. Acidity in closed and open tubes = glucose fermenter
2. Acidity in open tube only = glucose oxidizer
3. No acidity in either tube (neither glucose fermenter nor oxidizer) = inactive

Note:
Other carbohydrates may be incorporated into O-F medium to facilitate speciation of glucose oxidizers.

NONFERMENTING GRAM-NEGATIVE RODS

Recommended cultures to be studied: *P. aeruginosa, A. baumanii*, and *Moraxella* sp.

Instructions: Perform the following procedures for presumptive identification of *Pseudomonas* species, *Acinetobacter,* and *Moraxella* species.

1. Observe and examine the growth on blood agar, nutrient agar, and MacConkey agar.
2. Characterize any odor or pigmentation.
3. Inoculate an infusion agar slant and incubate at 42°C.
4. Prepare smears for Gram stain. Examine and describe the microscopic morphology.
5. Inoculate the following biochemical test media—TSI, citrate, motility—and oxidative-fermentative media—glucose, open and closed, maltose, lactose, xylose.
6. Perform an oxidase test on each organism.
7. Inoculate an API 20E or other miniaturized biochemical system.
8. Incubate all cultures for 18 to 24 hours at 37°C.
9. Read and record all results.

██████ LABORATORY WORKSHEET

NONFERMENTING GRAM-NEGATIVE RODS

Student Name _____

Date performed: _____
Date completed: _____

Colony Morphology

	Odor	Pigment
Pseudomonas sp		
Acinetobacter sp		
Moraxella sp		

Microscopic Morphology

Pseudomonas sp   *Acinetobacter* sp   *Moraxella* sp

Biochemical Test Results

Test/Results	Organisms		
	Pseudomonas	*Acinetobacter*	*Moraxella*
TSI			
Oxidase			
Citrate			
O-F glucose Open Closed			
Lactose			
Maltose			
Xylose			

CHAPTER 10

Miscellaneous Gram-Negative Rods

This chapter discusses the following genera of gram-negative bacilli: *Haemophilus, Bordetella, Brucella, Francisella,* and *Pasteurella. Brucella* and *Francisella* species are highly infectious agents, and therefore laboratory exercises do not include these organisms.

■■■■■ O B J E C T I V E S

1. Describe the characteristic colonial and microscopic morphology of the organisms previously listed.

2. List the nutritional and environmental growth requirements, if any, for these organisms.

3. List the primary isolation media used to cultivate these organisms.

4. Explain the proper specimen collection methods for cultivation of these organisms.

5. Give the biochemical test reactions used to identify or differentiate each species from other gram-negative organisms.

HAEMOPHILUS

Haemophilus are small, pleomorphic gram-negative rods that are common inhabitants of the upper respiratory tract. Given the proper conditions to colonize and become invasive in the appropriate hosts, however, these organisms are known to cause several serious infections. The most commonly encountered manifestations of *Haemophilus* infections include meningitis, acute bacterial epiglottitis, and septicemia. All species of *Haemophilus* require either one or both of special growth factors designated as X and V factors. X factor is a heat-stable factor, hemin, whereas V factor is heat-labile nicotinamide adenine dinucleotide (NAD). Chocolate agar is the culture medium commonly used to isolate *Haemophilus* species.

The following table shows the differential characteristics of *Haemophilus* species:

Species	Requires factors		Porphyrin	Hemolysis
	X	V		
H. influenzae	+	+	−	−
H. parainfluenzae	−	+	+	−
H. haemolyticus	+	+	−	+
H. parahaemolyticus	−	+	+	+
H. aphrophilus	−	−	+(weak)	−

BORDETELLA

There are three clinically significant species in the genus *Bordetella*: *B. pertussis,* causative agent of whooping cough; *B. parapertussis;* and *B. bronchoseptica.* These organisms are small, gram-negative coccobacilli and are strict aerobes. Although they do not require special growth factors as *Haemophilus* does, primary isolation does require a special culture medium (potato glycerol blood) with antimicrobials. These ingredients are added to neutralize any inhibitory effects of peroxides and unsaturated fatty acids. Antimicrobials are included to inhibit the growth of normal respiratory inhabitants. Colonies of *B. pertussis* on this medium appear smooth, convex, and pearl-like (mercury drops).

The following table shows the differentiating characteristics in the genus *Bordetella*:

Species	Growth on Heart Infusion Agar	Urease Nitrite Reduction	Motility
B. pertussis	−		−
B. parapertussis	+	+ (18 hours)	−
B. bronchoseptica	+	+ (4 hours)	+

PASTEURELLA

Pasteurella multocida is the most clinically significant species in this genus. These organisms are indigenous flora of animals, and therefore human infections are acquired through bites or scratch of a domestic dog or cat. *P. multocida* are small, gram-negative, pleomorphic coccobacilli. Similar to other *Pasteurella,* they show bipolar staining, giving a "safety pin" appearance microscopically. They grow well on sheep blood agar but not on MacConkey agar. *P. mutocida* ferment carbohydrates and are oxidase positive.

Aspirates of pus and occasionally sputum are the clinical samples from which these organisms are isolated.

X AND V STRIP IDENTIFICATION PROCEDURE FOR *HAEMOPHILUS*

Principle

The growth factors required by members of the genus *Haemophilus* are the heme portion of hemoglobin (X factor) and NAD (V factor). Differential identification of species within the genus may be made by determining the requirement for either one or both of the factors using commercially prepared paper disks impregnated with the factors and an unsupplemented medium for growth.

Equipment and Reagents

X factor strips (Difco or BBL); V factor strips; XV factor strips; Mueller-Hinton plate

Quality Control

Known control strains should be run with each group of tests performed.

Procedure

1. Obtain a heavy growth of the suspected *Haemophilus* isolate on chocolate agar, preferably a 24-hour culture.
2. Streak the suspected *Haemophilus* isolate over the entire surface of a Mueller-Hinton plate.
3. Place an X, V, and XV strip in the area of the inocula in three of the four quadrants. The fourth quadrant serves as a negative control.
4. Incubate the plate at 37°C under CO_2. Read for growth around disks at 24 hours.

Interpretation of Results

Growth around either one or both factor disks is interpreted as a requirement for that factor by the organism. Refer to Table on p. 103 for species requirements.

■■■■■■■   LABORATORY EXERCISE

MISCELLANEOUS GRAM-NEGATIVE RODS

Instructions:

1. Observe and examine colonial morphology of *H. influenzae,* *Bordetella,* and *Pasteurella multocida* on blood agar, chocolate agar, and MacConkey agar.
2. Prepare smears from each culture and Gram stain. Observe and describe the microscopic morphology of each organism.
3. Perform the following biochemical tests: Test *Haemophilus* sp for X and V factor requirements.

LABORATORY WORKSHEET

MISCELLANEOUS GRAM-NEGATIVE RODS

Student Name _____

Date performed: _____
Date completed: _____

Colony Morphology

Genus/Species	Blood Agar	Chocolate	MacConkey
Haemophilus sp			
Bordetella sp			
Pasteurella sp			

Microscopic Morphology

Haemophilus sp

Bordetella sp

Pasteurella sp

Biochemical Test Results

Haemophilus	Requires factors		Hemolysis (Casman's blood agar)
	X	V	
H. influenzae *H. parainfluenzae*			

CHAPTER 11

Medically Important Anaerobic Organisms

This chapter discusses medically significant anaerobic organisms such as *Veillonella, Clostridium* sp, *Bacteroides* species, and other anaerobic gram-negative bacilli.

■■■■■ O B J E C T I V E S

1. Describe the microscopic morphology of each of these species.

2. Discuss how the characteristic microscopic morphology of each representative organism may be used for presumptive identification of the isolate.

3. Describe characteristic colonial morphology of *Clostridium perfringens, Prevotella,* and *Porphyromonas*

species on blood containing agar medium and of *Bacteroides fragilis* on a selective medium such as BBE agar.

4. List the tests used to identify these species initially.

5. Presumptively identify *C. perfringens, Fusobacterium,* and *Bacteroides* species.

VEILLONELLA SPECIES

The genus *Veillonella* consists of anaerobic gram-negative cocci that are part of the normal oral flora and upper respiratory tract. Infections due to these organisms usually result from mucosal trauma. *Veillonella* produces small, convex translucent colonies on blood agar. Identification is made based on carbohydrate fermentation and fatty acid end products by gas liquid chromatography.

CLOSTRIDIUM

The genus *Clostridium* includes species that are widely distributed in nature. Several are members of the normal intestinal flora of both humans and animals. *Clostridium* is the only genus of gram-positive, anaerobic spore-forming bacilli that have been isolated from human clinical materials. One of the most important species, *C. perfringens,* causes gas gangrene and food-borne illness.

The Gram stain is an important diagnostic tool in recognizing the possibility of gas gangrene, supported by clinical diagnosis. The presence of large, short, fat, gram-positive bacilli in a direct smear from aspirated material should be regarded as a significant finding. *C. perfringens* colonies on blood agar plates show a double zone of hemolysis caused by two toxins produced by the organism. Other significant species are *Clostridium tetani, Clostridium botulinum,* and *Clostridium difficile.*

BACTEROIDES

Anaerobic gram-negative bacilli are members of the normal flora of the upper respiratory tract, intestinal tract, and the female genital tract. Therefore, infections associated with these organisms are opportunistic. The most commonly encountered pathogen in the clinical laboratory in the genus *Bacteroides* is *Bacteroides fragilis.* This capsulated, pale-staining, short, and slim gram-negative rod grows readily on blood agar medium. Resistance to 20% bile and resistance to special potency disk kanamycin are tests used to differentiate the species initially from other *Bacteroides* and *Fusobacterium.*

Formerly known as pigmented *Bacteroides,* members of the genera *Prevotella* and *Porphyromonas* are significant anaerobic species. These organisms are normal inhabitants of the mouth flora and are often associated with dental infections, pulmonary abscesses, and infections from human bites. Characteristic colonial morphology is the appearance of brick red fluorescence and black pigmented colonies when grown on blood agar medium. Bile sensitivity is used to identify these organisms initially.

FUSOBACTERIUM

Fusobacterium nucleatum and *Fusobacterium necrophorum* are two species of *Fusobacterium* most commonly encountered in the clinical laboratory. They are found as normal flora in the upper respiratory tract; therefore, resulting infections involve the head, neck, and lower respiratory tract. Members of the genus appear as long, slender, pale-staining gram-negative rods with tapered ends. Colonies on blood agar are usually nonhemolytic; appearance may vary from flat to convex with irregular margins. Growth in 20% bile is inhibited. Identification is characterized by large amounts of butyric acid produced as metabolic end product.

LABORATORY EXERCISE 1

CLOSTRIDIUM

Instructions: Recommended organisms to be studied are *C. perfringens* or any *Clostridium* species that demonstrates characteristic morphology of *Clostridium.*

1. Observe the growth of *C. perfringens* on blood agar plate. Describe the colonial appearance.
2. Prepare a smear from Gram stain.
3. Observe the microscopic morphology of the organism. Sketch a few cells.
4. The following tests may be performed or demonstrated. Observe and examine each test reaction and record results.
   ■ Cooked meat
   ■ Egg yolk agar
   ■ Litmus milk

▬▬▬▬▬   LABORATORY WORKSHEET

CLOSTRIDIUM

Student Name _____

Date performed: _____
Date completed: _____

Colony Morphology

	Description of Colonies
	C. perfringens
Blood agar	
KV agar	

Microscopic Morphology

C. perfringens
Gram stain _____
_____

Biochemical Test Results

Biochemical Reactions	Results
Litmus milk	
Cooked meat	
Egg yolk agar	

■■■■■■■ LABORATORY EXERCISE 2

ANAEROBIC GRAM-NEGATIVE RODS

Instructions: Recommended organisms to be studied (if available) include:

- *B. fragilis*
- *Fusobacterium*
- *Prevotella*
- *Porphyromonas*

1. Observe and examine colonial morphology of *B. fragilis,*
Prevotella sp or *Porphyromonas* sp
   - Blood agar
   - KV
   - BBE agar
2. Prepare smears from each culture and Gram stain.
3. Describe the microscopic morphology of each culture.
4. Other tests that may be performed or demonstrated include special potency disks susceptibility.

■■■■■■■   LABORATORY WORKSHEET

ANAEROBIC GRAM-NEGATIVE RODS

Student Name _____

Date performed: _____
Date completed: _____

Colony Morphology

Culture Medium	Description of Colonies		
Blood agar KV agar BBE agar			

Microscopic Morphology

CHAPTER 12

Medically Important Fungi and Mycobacteria

Mycobacteria and fungi are organisms that are seen infrequently and usually require a more extensive work-up, including prolonged incubation times; thus, most medical technologists who work in a clinical laboratory feel uncomfortable working with these organisms. In the past few years, however, these organisms have been seen in increasing numbers as causes of significant disease in the immunocompromised host.

Procedures for collection and processing of clinical samples for the recovery of mycobacteria and fungi are described in Chapters 22 and 23, *Textbook of Diagnostic Microbiology*.

OBJECTIVES

1. Observe the defined structures for identification of selected fungal agents demonstrated in the following preparations:

   - KOH preparation of a skin scraping
   - India ink preparation
   - Lactophenol cotton blue preparation

2. Perform the following procedures to presumptively identify yeast species:

   - Germ tube test
   - Wet mount preparation—yeast

3. Prepare a smear for acid-fast bacillus stain. Observe the morphology of an acid-fast bacillus stained with Ziehl-Neelsen or Kinyoun AFB staining method.

GERM TUBE TEST

Principle

The germ tube test is a screening procedure for *Candida albicans* and *Candida stellatoidea*. Germ tubes are readily formed by most strains of both. *C. stellatoidea* is rare, however.

Specimen Requirements

Pure yeast colony from culture slant or plate.

Quality Control

- Positive Control = *C. albicans*
- Negative control = *Candida tropicalis*

Reagents

Sterile Fetal Bovine Serum; Dessicated Fetal Calf Serum— Serum is reconstituted and stored in premeasured 0.5-mL aliquots in freezer. Thaw as needed. Do not refreeze.

Equipment and Supplies

1. Microscope
2. Sterile pasteur pipettes
3. Incubator, 37°C
4. Clean glass slides
5. Coverslips (22 × 22 mm)
6. 13 × 100 mm sterile test tubes

Procedure

1. Pick a yeast colony with a pasteur pipette (a small amount on end of pipette is sufficient).
2. Mix yeast cells in 0.5 mL fetal bovine serum in 10 × 75 mm test tube. Include controls.
3. Place tube with pipette in 37°C incubator for 2 hours.
4. Use pipette to transfer one drop to a clean slide, coverslip, and examine for presence of germ tubes.

Results

Observed microscopically, a germ tube appears as an extension from the yeast cell: This tube has parallel sides with no constriction as it leaves the cell. Pseudohyphae does not have parallel sides, and may be septate.

If germ tube test is positive, the yeast isolate can be presumptively identified as *C. albicans*.

Notes:

1. *Germ tubes may not form in some rare strains of C. albicans.*
2. *Test should be examined within 3 hours because C. tropicalis develops pseudohyphae after that length of time.*
3. *Gross bacterial contamination may inhibit the induction of germ tubes.*

WET-MOUNT PREPARATION

Principle

Direct microscopic examination of clinical specimens for microorganisms is extremely important. It provides immediate information on the mature and relative numbers of various microbial organisms, inflammatory and other host cells, and certain other materials, such as crystals.

It is often necessary to examine certain microorganisms in the living state because they are not readily stained or because they cannot be easily cultivated. Also, when they are examined in the living state, morphology is less distorted, and motility and other characteristics may be observed readily.

Reagents

Physiologic saline 0.89%—Store at room temperature; expires as dated. Distilled water.

Procedure

There are two approaches, the choice being determined by the nature of the specimens.

1. Place a loopful of liquid clinical specimen or culture on a clean glass slide and cover with a coverglass.
2. Or place a loopful of clean water on the slide, emulsify some nonliquid clinical material or portion of a bacterial colony in it, and add a coverglass.
3. Examine the preparation immediately before the liquid starts to evaporate.

Results

Specimens received in the laboratory for microbiologic examination can vary widely. Wet-mount preparations may be used to look for particular organisms such as saline wet-mount preparations for *Trichomonas* and direct mounts for ameba, ova, and other parasites and yeasts.

POTASSIUM HYDROXIDE (KOH) PREPARATION

Principle

KOH mounting fluid is used mainly for the examination of skin, nails, and hair for the presence of fungal elements. The hydroxide solution serves as a cleaning agent, and the heating hastens its actions.

Specimen

Any clinical material may be used (pus, fluids, exudate, tissue), most often skin, hair, or nail scrapings or fragments.

Reagents

10% KOH

Reagent Preparation

To prepare, weigh 10 g of KOH. Dissolve slowly in 100 mL distilled water.

Quality Control

The procedure provides its own control. KOH solution may be checked by mounting a hair fragment and observing for cleaning action.

Procedure

1. Place a drop of 10% KOH in the center of a clean glass slide.
2. Wet teasing needle in KOH.
3. Pick up clinical material with needle. Use several pieces of material if available. Tease material to give a thin preparation.
4. Mount the coverslip over the material and gently heat the preparation by passing it through a Bunsen burner flame two or three times.
5. Spread material out by gently pressing it with the butt end of the teasing needle on the coverslip. Let it stand for 5 minutes and, if material is not flat, press again.
6. Examine the preparation microscopically under low power and confirm the observations under high power. If the preparation is not thin enough, allow it to sit for 15 minutes and then examine. Two or three hours may be required to soften nail scrapings sufficiently to spread them out for microscopic examination.

Expected Results

Examine for any hyphae and other fungal elements.

Infected skin and nail scrapings show saline, septate, branching hyphae, and arthroconidia.

Infected hairs show hyphae in the interior of the hair shaft or outside the hair shaft.

Report Format:

1. No fungal elements observed
2. Fungal structures present: (name structures observed)

Notes:
KOH-negative specimens may yield positive cultures.

INDIA INK PREPARATIONS

Principle

The capsule of microorganisms does not have the same affinity for dyes as do other cell components, which necessitates the use of a special staining procedure.

In the India ink method, the capsule displaces the colloidal carbon particles of the ink and appears as a clean halo around the microorganism. The procedure is especially recommended for demonstrating the capsule of *Cryptococcus neoformans*.

Specimen Requirement

1. Culture of the organism to be tested
2. Cerebrospinal fluid

Reagent

Pelikan India ink—store at room temperature.

Procedure

1. To a small loopful of saline or water on a clean slide, add a minute amount of growth from a young agar culture, using an inoculating needle.

   Spinal fluid may be used directly.
2. Mix well, then add a small loopful of India ink and immediately cover with a thin coverglass, allowing the fluid to spread as a thin film beneath the coverglass.
3. Examine immediately under the oil immersion objective, reducing the light considerably by lowering the condenser. Capsules, when present, stand out as clean halos against a dark background.

ZIEHL-NEELSEN ACID-FAST STAIN

Principle

Ziehl-Neelsen differential stain is used to separate acid-fast organisms from non–acid-fast organisms. Mycobacteria resist decolorization by acid or alcohol and are therefore called "acid-fast" bacilli. Phenol is used as a mordant, fuchsin as a dye, and acid-alcohol as a decolorizing agent. Counterstain with brilliant green or methylene blue.

Specimen Requirement

Prepare smear by spreading a drop of inoculum (concentrated sediment or suspension of organism from a culture) over an area 2 to 3 cm on a slide.

Reagents

1. Carbol-fuchsin
   ■ Saturated alcoholic solution of basic fuchsin (3 g basic fuchsin in 100 mL of 95% ethyl alcohol)—10.0 mL
   ■ 5% aqueous solution of phenol (weigh 5.0 g phenol crystals, melt with gentle heat, add 100 mL H_2O—90.0 mL
2. Acid-alcohol
   ■ HCL (conc.)—3.0 mL
   ■ Ethyl alcohol (95%)—97.0 mL
3. Counterstain
   ■ Methylene blue chloride—0.3 g
   ■ Distilled water—100.0 mL

The aforementioned reagents are commercially available.

Quality Control

■ Positive control = *Mycobacterium* sp
■ Negative control = *Escherichia coli*

Equipment and Supplies

1. Microscope slides, frosted end
2. Sterile Pasteur pipettes
3. Slide warmer, 65°C
4. Slide staining rack
5. Timing clock
6. Tap water
7. Microscope with oil immersion lens
8. Immersion oil
9. Electric staining bath

Procedure

1. Turn staining bath heat control knob to "high" and allow to warm up for at least 15 minutes.
2. Prepare smears and heat fix on slide warmer for 2 hours at 65°C.

3. Place smears on staining rack on electric staining bath. Flood smears with carbol-fuchsin. Allow to stand for 5 to 10 minutes. (More carbol-fuchsin may need to be added during heating process.)

4. Remove staining rack from top of staining bath and place over sink. Rinse slides with tap water.

5. Decolorize in two steps.
   - Decolorize for 1 minute; rinse with tap water.
   - Repeat decolorizer for 1 minute; rinse slides with tap water.

6. Counterstain for 1 minute with brilliant green or methylene blue.

7. Wash with tap water. Air dry. Do not blot.

8. Examine smear with oil immersion lens, taking care to wipe the lens well after each slide. Three long lines the length of the smear or nine short lines the width of the smear are examined.

Results

Acid-fast bacilli are stained red, and the background and non—acid-fast organisms are stained blue or green. Reports should state the number of acid-fast bacilli seen on the smear. Report as follows:

Number of bacilli	Report
0	No acid-fast bacilli seen
1–2 in entire smear	Report number found
3–9 in entire smear	Rare
10 or more in entire smear	Few
1 or more per field	Numerous

■■■■■■■ LABORATORY EXERCISE 1

MYCOBACTERIA AND COMMONLY ENCOUNTERED MOLDS

Instructions: Because of the biohazard nature of these agents, it is recommended that all laboratory exercises be carried out with extreme caution. It is also suggested that identification of these agents be presented as a demonstration exercise.

Recommended cultures to be studied:

- *Mycobacteria—Mycobacterium* species (QC positive and negative slides)
- *Fungal agents* (prepared slides of the following fungal species): *Alternaria, Curvularia, Rhizopus* sp, *Mucor* sp, *Aspergillus, Penicillium, Microsporum gypseum,* *Microsporum canis, Trichophyton rubrum, Trichophyton mentagrophytes, Epidermophyton floccusum, Sporothrix schenckii*
- *Blastomyces dermatitidis* (if available)
- *Histoplasma capsulatum* subsp *capsulatum* (if available)
- *Coccidioides immitis* (if available)

1. Observe the colonial morphology of the above-mentioned fungal cultures and microscopic morphology in lactophenol cotton blue preparations.
2. Observe the diagnostic microscopic structures for each species.

LABORATORY WORKSHEET

MYCOBACTERIA AND COMMONLY ENCOUNTERED MOLDS

Sketch a few cells demonstrating the characteristic morphology of prepared smears:

Worksheet continued on following page

MYCOBACTERIA AND COMMONLY ENCOUNTERED MOLDS

Sketch a few cells demonstrating the characteristic morphology of prepared smears:

Worksheet continued on opposite page

■■■■■■ LABORATORY WORKSHEET *Continued*

MYCOBACTERIA AND COMMONLY ENCOUNTERED MOLDS

Sketch a few cells demonstrating the characteristic morphology of prepared smears:

■■■■■■■■   LABORATORY EXERCISE 2

YEASTS

Instructions: Recommended cultures to be studied:

- ■ *Candida albicans*
- ■ *Candida tropicalis*
- ■ *Candida pseudotropicalis*

1. Observe the gross colonial morphology of the above-mentioned organisms on blood agar medium and on Sabouraud's dextrose agar and the microscopic morphology on cornmeal Tween 80 agar.
2. Make a sketch of morphology observed on each species.
3. Perform germ tube test on the above-mentioned organisms and record the results.
4. Perform or demonstrate assimilation tests (optional).

LABORATORY WORKSHEET

YEASTS

Student Name _____

Date performed: _____
Date completed: _____

Colony Morphology on Sabouraud's Dextrose Agar and Blood Agar

	Sabouraud's Dextrose Agar	Blood Agar
Candida albicans		
Candida tropicalis		
Candida pseudotropicalis		

Worksheet continued on following page

Microscopic Morphology on Cornmeal Tween 80 Agar

Morphology

Candida albicans	
Candida tropicalis	
Candida pseudotropicalis	

Germ Tube Test	Results/Comments
Candida albicans	
Candida tropicalis	
Candida pseudotropicalis	

Laboratory Diagnosis of
Infectious Diseases

CHAPTER 13

Etiologic Agents Encountered in Infectious Diseases

This chapter discusses the different bacterial agents commonly encountered from clinical samples submitted to the microbiology laboratory for diagnosis of infectious diseases. Interpretation of culture results from respiratory, genitourinary, and intestinal tracts is covered.

■■■■ OBJECTIVES

1. Assess the suitability of the clinical samples for microbiologic studies.

2. Given a clinical sample from a particular body site, differentiate organisms that are normal flora from those that are potential pathogens.

3. Identify the pathogenic organism present in a given sample.

4. Correctly report the results from the work-up of a specimen.

UPPER RESPIRATORY TRACT

Throat

The normal flora of the upper respiratory tract in healthy individuals consists of the following organisms:

- Nonhemolytic streptococci
- Staphylococci
- Micrococci
- *Corynebacterium* species
- *Neisseria* species
- *Veillonella* species

Routine throat cultures should be examined for the presence of group A streptococcus. Any growth in large amounts of potential pathogens such as *Staphylococcus aureus, Candida albicans,* and *Streptococcus pneumoniae* should be reported. If culture for *Bordetella pertussis* is specifically requested, plate to appropriate media and report the presence or absence accordingly.

Sputum

The following organisms are likely to be isolated and may be identified by colonial morphology. Report these organisms as "normal flora," and do not quantitate individually unless the growth is confluent with one organism.

- α-Hemolytic streptococci
- Diphtheroids
- Nonhemolytic streptococci
- *Staphylococcus epidermidis*
- *Neisseria* sp

Report the identification of the following organisms and perform suscepti-bility studies where applicable:

- *S. aureus* (moderate-to-heavy growth)
- Group A β hemolytic streptococcus
- *S. pneumoniae*
- *Haemophilus influenzae*
- *Corynebacterium diphtheriae*
- Gram-negative rod or enterococci
- Yeasts

Transtracheal Aspirates

Transtracheal aspirates are most useful in the diagnosis of pneumonia caused by aerobic or anaerobic organisms. The aspirate is obtained by percuta-neous needle entry into the trachea below the larynx, thereby avoiding contami-nation of lung aspirates with normal throat flora. Identify *any organisms* from transtracheal aspirates and do appropriate susceptibility studies.

Nose and Nasopharyngeal Cultures

Apply the same criteria as for sputum cultures. Carefully examine nasopha-ryngeal specimens for the presence of *Neisseria meningitidis* and *H. influenzae*.

Sinus and Mastoid Cultures

Apply the same criteria used for nasopharyngeal cultures.

Ear and Eye Cultures

Organisms not requiring complete identifications include:

- Diphtheroids
- *S. epidermidis*
- Viridans streptococci

The most commonly encountered pathogens that should be identified and sensi-tivity tested if appropriate are:

- *H. influenzae*

- *S. pneumoniae*
- Group A or β-hemolytic streptococci
- *S. aureus*
- *Pseudomonas aeruginosa*
- *Neisseria gonorrhoeae* (from eye culture)
- Yeasts

GENITOURINARY TRACT

Urine Cultures

The following semiquantitative counts are considered significant. Identification and appropriate susceptibilities should be performed:

- <100,000 org/mL of a pure culture
- 50,000 of each of two organisms
- 10,000 to 100,000 org/mL of a pure culture
- 100,000 org/mL of two organisms; list the approximate count of each of the organisms identified

Up to three different species regardless of the count are likely to be significant on the following specimens:

- Catheterized urine samples
- Cystoscopy specimens from the ureters, bladder, or kidney
- Suprapubic taps
- Bladder aspirates
- Post–kidney transplant patients
- Patients with renal calculi (stones)
- Paraplegics

Genital Cultures

Cervical, vaginal, or urethral cultures for detection of gonorrhea are cultured on Thayer-Martin and incubated under CO_2 for a total of 72 hours. Report "no *N. gonorrhoeae* isolated in 72 hours" or "oxidase-positive, gram-negative diplococci isolated, morphologically and biochemically consistent with *N. gonorrhoeae*."

For vaginal cultures, identify and do sensitivities where applicable on the following organisms with or without the presence of usual vaginal flora:

- *N. gonorrhoeae*
- *Listeria monocytogenes*
- *S. aureus*
- β-hemolytic streptococci, group A or B
- *Gardnerella vaginalis*

- Moderate-to-heavy growth of a gram-negative rod or enterococcus
- Yeasts

Abscesses or surgically obtained specimens of endometrium, fallopian tubes, and so forth are cultured for anaerobes as well as aerobes.

AEROBIC EXUDATE AND WOUND CULTURES

Organisms most frequently isolated that require identification and appropriate sensitivities include:

- *S. aureus*
- *β*-hemolytic streptococci
- *Pseudomonas* sp
- Enterococci
- Enteric bacilli

Other organisms less frequently isolated but highly significant are:

- *C. diphtheriae*
- *Bacillus anthracis*
- *Erysipelothrix rhusiopathiae*

ANAEROBIC CULTURES OF ABSCESSES

All organisms in a properly collected sample of a closed abscess are potentially significant. Therefore, all organisms should be identified. Susceptibility testing may be done on request. Most frequently expected pathogens include:

- *Bacteroides* sp
- *Clostridium* sp (especially *C. perfringens*)
- Anaerobic gram-positive cocci

TOOTH ABSCESSES AND OTHER CULTURES OF THE MOUTH

Tooth abscesses appear often to be caused by a mixture of both aerobic and anaerobic bacteria, which collectively constitute usual mouth flora. Unfortunately, collection procedures rarely allow differentiation of normal flora from infecting organisms. Therefore, report the results of such cultures as follows:

1. Identify and report *S. aureus* or *β*-hemolytic streptococci.
2. Report a heavy or predominant growth of a yeast.
3. Report the presence of a pure culture or a mixture of only two organisms.
4. Report a mixture of three or more normal flora organisms as "usual mouth flora."

Use the same criteria for reporting the results of any other culture of material from the mouth.

INTESTINAL TRACT

The normal flora of the intestinal tract contains both aerobes and anaerobes, with anaerobes outnumbering aerobes by 1000 to 1. Intestinal pathogens may include:

- *Salmonella*
- *Shigella*
- *Vibrio cholerae*
- *Yersinia enterocolitica*
- *Vibrio parahaemolyticus*
- Some strains of *Escherichia coli*
- *Clostridium difficile* (toxin)
- *Campylobacter* species

███████   LABORATORY WORKSHEET

ETIOLOGIC AGENTS IN INFECTIOUS DISEASES

Instructions:

1. For the following clinical samples, isolate and identify significant organisms cultured. Perform only the necessary tests and procedures.
   - Sputum
   - Urine
   - Throat
   - Stool

2. Perform susceptibility studies when applicable.
3. Report only significant isolates and "normal flora" when applicable.
4. Record all biochemical, macroscopic, and microscopic description on isolates.
5. Record all results on the laboratory worksheets provided.

███████   S P E C I M E N: _____

Colonial Morphology: Isolate # _____ BAP Choc Mac HE XLD **Gram Stain:**	Biochemical Tests	Identification
Report:		
Colonial Morphology: Isolate # _____ BAP Choc Mac HE XLD **Gram Stain:**		
Report:		

Exercise continued on opposite page

■■■■■ LABORATORY WORKSHEET *Continued*

ETIOLOGIC AGENTS IN INFECTIOUS DISEASES

■■■■ S P E C I M E N: _____

Colonial Morphology: Isolate # _____ BAP Choc Mac HE XLD Gram Stain:	Biochemical Tests	Identification
Report:		
Colonial Morphology: Isolate # _____ BAP Choc Mac HE XLD Gram Stain:		
Report:		

■■■■ S P E C I M E N: _____

Colonial Morphology: Isolate # _____ BAP Choc Mac HE XLD Gram Stain:	Biochemical Tests	Identification
Report:		
Colonial Morphology: Isolate # _____ BAP Choc Mac HE XLD Gram Stain:		
Report:		

Exercise continued on following page

■■■■■   LABORATORY WORKSHEET *Continued*

ETIOLOGIC AGENTS IN INFECTIOUS DISEASES

■■■■■   S P E C I M E N: _____

Colonial Morphology: Isolate # _____
    BAP
    Choc
    Mac
    HE
    XLD
Gram Stain:
	Biochemical Tests	Identification

Report:		

Colonial Morphology: Isolate # _____
    BAP
    Choc
    Mac
    HE
    XLD
Gram Stain:		

Report:		

■■■■■   S P E C I M E N: _____

Colonial Morphology: Isolate # _____
    BAP
    Choc
    Mac
    HE
    XLD
Gram Stain:
	Biochemical Tests	Identification

Report:		

Colonial Morphology: Isolate # _____
    BAP
    Choc
    Mac
    HE
    XLD
Gram Stain:		

Report:		

CHAPTER 14

Antimicrobial Susceptibility Testing

This chapter consists of procedures for performing and interpreting the following antimicrobial susceptibility tests: Kirby-Bauer disk diffusion, macrodilution broth, and serum antimicrobial activity.

■■■■■ O B J E C T I V E S

1. Explain the principles of the following susceptibility testing procedures:

   ■ Kirby-Bauer
   ■ Macrodilution minimal inhibitory concentration
   ■ Serum antimicrobial activity or Schlicter test

2. Perform susceptibility testing using the Kirby-Bauer disk diffusion method.

3. Determine minimal inhibitory concentration by the macrodilution susceptibility test.

4. List the elements that are significant in achieving accurate and reproducible results when performing susceptibility tests.

5. Discuss the effect of change in the following components of the test:
   ■ Medium
   ■ pH
   ■ Inoculum density
   ■ Incubator temperature

6. Discuss the limitations of each of the above-mentioned procedures.

7. Describe the clinical applications and the significance of serum antimicrobial activity (Schlicter test) and serum bactericidal levels.

KIRBY-BAUER DISK DIFFUSION SUSCEPTIBILITY TESTING PROCEDURE

Antimicrobial susceptibility tests are used to determine susceptibility or resistance of a pathogenic organism to a particular antimicrobial agent. Standardized paper disks impregnated with known amounts of antimicrobials are used to measure the susceptibility of microorganisms to these agents. The standardized disk susceptibility test, which is a modification of the test described by Bauer, Kirby, Sherris, and Turck, is recommended for clinical laboratories.

With the exception of a few organisms such as group A β-streptococci, susceptibility test is performed routinely on all clinically significant isolates. Organisms that are considered usual flora of a particular anatomic site are not tested. These include α-streptococci, *Neisseria* sp, and diphtheroids (not *C. diphtheriae*) from the throat and expectorated sputum and *Escherichia coli, Enterobacter* sp, *Klebsiella* sp, and *Proteus* sp from rectal and stool cultures. Special procedures in performing susceptibility tests on fastidious organisms are described in Chapter 3B, *Textbook of Diagnostic Microbiology*.

Some of the commonly used antimicrobials for testing against certain groups of bacteria are listed as follows:

1. Gram-positive bacteria:
   - Ampicillin
   - Gentamicin
   - Cephalosporin
   - Clindamycin
   - Erythromycin
   - Tetracycline
   - Oxacillin
   - Penicillin G
2. Gram-negative bacteria:
   - Ampicillin
   - Cephalosporin
   - Tetracycline
   - Trimethoprim/sulfamethoxazole
   - Ticarcillin
   - Gentamicin
3. *Pseudomonas aeruginosa* isolates:
   - Amikacin
   - Gentamicin
   - Tobramycin
   - Ticarcillin
   - Piperacillin

In performing Kirby-Bauer susceptibility tests, the procedure must be strictly followed, including preparation of media and inocula. Factors such as incubation temperature and environmental conditions may also affect interpretive results.

There are several factors that may affect zone size interpretations, hence "false susceptible" or "false resistant" results may occur. Table 14–1 shows some of the factors that may affect zone size interpretations.

MACRODILUTION BROTH PROCEDURE FOR THE DETERMINATION OF MINIMAL INHIBITORY CONCENTRATION

The minimal inhibitory concentration (MIC) of an antimicrobial is performed on clinically significant organisms isolated from serious infections; from infections that require long antimicrobial therapy, such as subacute bacterial endocarditis and osteomyelitis; from infections in body sites where attainable levels are low, such as cerebrospinal fluid and biliary tract; or from fastidious or slow-growing organisms that cannot be tested with the Kirby-Bauer method.

Diagnostic reagent powder is used and dissolved in the appropriate solvent. The antimicrobial agent is then diluted to appropriate concentrations in broth. A standard inoculum of the organism is added in equal volume to each of the concentration of antimicrobial agent. The lowest concentration of the antimicrobial agent that inhibits growth of the organism is designated as MIC.

■■■■■ T A B L E   14 – 1

FACTORS THAT MAY AFFECT ZONE SIZE INTERPRETATIONS

Effects of	Result	Action to Be Taken
pH of medium		
Too low	Tetracycline zone too large; clindamycin too small with *E. coli* and *S. aureus* controls	Adjust pH to 7.2–7.4 before pouring
		Commercial media usually have right pH
Too high	Tetracycline zone too small; clindamycin too large with *E. coli* and *S. aureus*	Get a new lot; CO_2 may alter surface pH
Ca^{++} and Mg^{++}		
Too high	Aminoglycoside zone too small with *P. aeruginosa*	Acquire a new lot
Too low	Aminoglycoside zone too large with *P. aeruginosa*	Acquire a new lot
Inoculum density		
Too light	All zone sizes too large on control organism	Adjust to McFarland 0.5 turbidity standard
Too heavy	All zone sizes too small on control organisms	Same as above
Depth of the agar		
Too thin	All zone sizes too large on control organisms	Use 4–5 mm depth
Too thick	All zone sizes too small on control organisms	
Storage	Methicillin zone decreases over days with control organisms	Methicillin degrades during refrigerator storage. Change methicillin disks

If the MIC can be readily achieved in the patient's serum by normal routes, the organism is said to be "susceptible."

DETERMINATION OF SERUM ANTIMICROBIAL ACTIVITY

The test for serum antimicrobial activity or Schlicter test provides a semi-quantitative data (minimal bactericidal dilution or MBD) concerning the ability of the patient's serum to kill his or her own infecting organism in situations in which the patient is not responding to the antimicrobial therapy. This test also determines if the level of antimicrobial therapy is adequate to inhibit or kill the patient's own infecting organism in critical clinical conditions, such as subacute bacterial endocarditis, osteomyelitis, and septicemia.

■■■■■■■   LABORATORY EXERCISE 1

KIRBY-BAUER SUSCEPTIBILITY TEST

Instructions:

1. Using quality control organisms and a patient unknown, perform the Kirby-Bauer test following the procedure outlined:
   - *E. coli* ATCC 25922
   - *S. aureus* ATCC 25923
   - *P. aeruginosa* ATCC 27853
   - Patient unknown
2. After 18 hours of incubation, measure the zone size diameters and record on the worksheets provided. Indicate if the test organism is "susceptible," "intermediate," or "resistant" to each of the antimicrobial tested.
3. Compare your results with the expected results listed in the most updated interpretive zone diameters found in package inserts of antimicrobial disks.

Inoculum

1. Select three to five similar-appearing isolated colonies. Touch the top of each colony with a loop and transfer this inoculum to 1 mL of trypticase soy broth.
2. Incubate the broth at 35°C for a minimum of 1 hour to produce an organism suspension with light cloudiness, which approximates the McFarland 0.5 standard.
3. Dilute the growth if necessary with sterile water to obtain the necessary turbidity.

Streaking Plates

1. Use 150-mm Mueller-Hinton agar plates for performance of the test.
2. Dip a sterile swab into the inoculum. Remove the excess inoculum from the swab by rotating it several times with firm pressure against the inside wall of the test tube above the fluid level.
3. Inoculate the entire sterile agar surface of the plate by streaking successively on three different axes to obtain an even inoculum.
4. Replace the plate top and allow the inoculum to dry for 3 to 5 minutes before applying the disks.
5. Disks are applied to the inoculated agar surface with the disk dispenser. Gently press each disk with sterile forceps to ensure even contact with the agar. Because diffusion of the drug is almost instantaneous, a disk should not be moved once it has come in contact with the agar surface.
6. Within 30 minutes, after the disks have been applied, place the plates in the 35°C incubator without CO_2.

Reading the Plates

1. Plates are incubated for 18 to 24 hours. Growth on the plates should be confluent. If isolated colonies are present, the inoculum was too light and the test must be repeated.
2. Measure the diameter of each zone of complete inhibition to the nearest whole millimeter using a ruler.
3. The end points are taken as the area showing no macroscopically visible growth.
4. When swarming is encountered with *Proteus* sp, measure the most obvious zones of growth and do not consider an area of swarming as indicative of resistance.

Interpretation of Zone Diameters

Report the results of susceptibility tests according to the most updated interpretive zone diameters found in package inserts of antimicrobial disks.

LABORATORY WORKSHEET

KIRBY-BAUER SUSCEPTIBILITY TEST

Student Name _____

Date performed: _____
Date completed: _____

■■■■■■■   LABORATORY EXERCISE 2

MACRODILUTION PROCEDURE

Instructions: Follow the procedure described:

1. Determine the MIC of penicillin against *S. epidermidis.*
2. Perform the procedure for determining the minimal bacteri-cidal level (MBC).
3. Determine if the MIC will provide a "susceptible" or "resis-tant" result.

Preparation of Antimicrobial Solution in Broth

1. Thaw the frozen stock solution of the antimicrobial and dilute it in sterile distilled water to a concentration that is 20 times the initial test concentration.
2. Label two sets of 12 tubes (tube #1 to #12).
3. Place 1.8/mL of Mueller-Hinton broth into tube #1 and 1.0 mL of Mueller-Hinton broth into tubes #2 to #12.
4. Add 0.2 mL of the diluted antimicrobial to tube #1, making a 1:10 dilution.
5. Continue with twofold serial dilutions of the antimicrobial by transferring 1.0 mL from tube #1 to the next consecutive tube, thoroughly mixing each dilution. See example.
6. Repeat the procedure for the next nine tubes (#3 to #10).
7. Discard 1.0 mL from tube #10.

Preparation of Inoculum

1. Select three to five similar-looking colonies.
2. Inoculate 5.0 mL of trypticase soy broth with the selected colonies.
3. Incubate for 2 to 5 hours. Adjust the density of the inoculum suspension to the turbidity of the 0.5 #1 McFarland standard using 0.9% sterile saline.

Inoculation of the Medium

1. Add 0.05 mL of diluted inoculum suspension to each tube (tube #1 to #11). Do not add any inoculum suspension to the negative control.
2. Add the inoculum just below the surface of the medium. Do not shake the inoculated medium.
3. Label two separate tubes 1:10 and 1:100 and place 0.9 mL of Mueller-Hinton broth. To the tube (1:10), add 0.1 mL of the *inoculated positive control.* Mix thoroughly.
4. Transfer 0.1 mL from the 1:10 dilution to the 1:100 dilu-tion. Mix.
5. Label two separate blood agar plates with 1:10 and 1:100

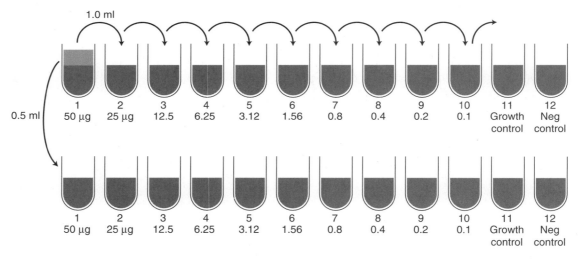

8. Transfer 0.5 mL from each tube to the second set of tubes, which serves as quality control.
9. Tube #11 serves as growth control and tube #12 as negative control.

dilution. Using 10-μL pipette, inoculate and streak the respec-tive plate from the 1:10 and 1:100 dilution.
6. Incubate all tubes and the two agar plates for 18 to 24 hours.

Exercise continued on opposite page

MACRODILUTION PROCEDURE

Results

1. The lowest concentration of antimicrobic resulting in complete inhibition of visible growth represents MIC.
2. Report the MIC in μg/mL of the particular drug.
3. Examine the blood agar plates containing the 1:10 and 1:100 dilution of the inoculum. Count the approximate number of colonies on each plate and multiply by 1000 for the 1:10 dilution and 10,000 for the 1:100 dilution.
4. The resulting number indicates the number of organisms per milliliter at the start of the test. For example:

$$1:10 \text{ dilution} = 20 \text{ colonies}$$

$$20 \times 10 \ (100 \text{ mL}) = 200{,}000 \text{ or } 2 \times 10^5$$

Determination of the Minimal Bactericidal Concentration

1. Shake all clear tubes after 18 to 20 hours of incubation, then reincubate at 35°C for 4 more hours before subculture.
2. Using a 10-μL pipette, subculture each of the negative-appearing tubes and the first tube that shows visible growth onto agar plates.
3. Streak inoculum over entire surface of the plate.
4. Incubate the subculture plates for 18 to 24 hours at 35°C.
5. Examine the plates for the presence of growth of the test organism. Count the number of colonies present.
6. Calculate the MBC (the least concentration of the antimicrobic that kills 99.9% of the organisms under the test conditions).

LABORATORY WORKSHEET

MACRODILUTION (MIC) PROCEDURE

Student Name _____

Date performed: _____
Date completed: _____

SCHLICTER TEST

Instructions: This procedure may be demonstrated or performed by students. Following the procedure described:

1. Perform Schlicter test on the following samples:
   ■ Predose serum sample
   ■ Postdose serum sample
2. Record results on the worksheets provided.
3. Determine the serum inhibitory titer and serum bactericidal titer obtained from each sample.

Serum Specimen Preparation

1. Collect 10 mL of blood in a sterile red top tube just before the next antimicrobial dose. This is the trough level. Thirty minutes postdose, collect a second 10-mL red top tube. This is the peak level.
2. Separate the serum and freeze at −20°C if the test is not run immediately.
3. Prepare twofold serial dilutions of the patient's serum.
   ■ Label 11 tubes (tube #1 to #11).
   ■ Place 0.5 mL of pooled serum to tubes #2 to #10 .
   ■ Add 0.5 mL of the patient's serum to tubes #1 (undiluted) and #2 (1 : 2 dilution).
   ■ Using a different pipette each time, mix and transfer 0.5 mL from tube #2 to tube #3.
   ■ Continue in this manner through tube #8 (1 : 128 dilution) discarding 0.5 mL from the last tube.
   ■ Tube #9 is negative control containing 0.5 mL pooled serum and 0.5 mL Mueller-Hinton broth (to be added in the next step). Tube #10 is a positive control containing 0.5 mL pooled serum, 0.5 mL Mueller-Hinton broth, and the inoculum. Tube #11 is the patient serum control containing 0.5 mL Mueller-Hinton broth and 0.5 mL patient's serum.
   ■ Add 0.5 mL of supplemented Mueller-Hinton broth to all tubes. The tubes now contain 50% serum and 50% broth, which further dilutes the mixture by half.
   ■ The final dilution for each tube is shown below:

Patient Culture Preparation

1. Inoculate the patient's organism into 10 mL of Mueller-Hinton broth and incubate 18 to 24 hours at 37°C.
2. Prepare a 1 :1000 dilution of the broth culture of the organism according to the following technique.
   a. Label three test tubes (#1–#3).
   b. Add 4.5 mL of casein soy broth to all tubes.
   c. Add 0.5 mL of the culture to tube #1.
   d. Mix and transfer 0.5 mL of the mixture from tube #1 to tube #2.
   e. Mix and transfer 0.5 mL of the mixture from tube #2 to the third tube of 4.5 mL of casein soy broth to obtain a 1:1000 dilution.

Inoculation of Diluted Serum Sample

1. Add 0.1 mL of the 1:1000 dilution of the broth culture of the organism to tubes #1 to #8 and tube #10.
2. Incubate all tubes for 18 to 24 hours at 37°C.
3. After 18 hours of incubation, examine each tube for visible growth.

The bacteriostatic level or maximal inhibitory dilution (MID) or serum inhibitory titer (SIT) is the highest dilution showing no visible growth. Be sure to check that there is no growth on the control tubes (tubes #9 and #11) and that there is growth on culture tube #10.

4. Plate the contents of all tubes with no visible growth to blood agar plates. Use a wire loop and do not touch the sides of the tube. Avoid splattering.
5. Incubate overnight at 37°C.
6. The highest dilution showing no growth is the MBD or serum bactericidal titer (SBT).

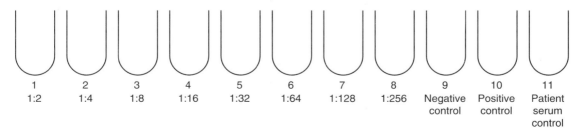

1	2	3	4	5	6	7	8	9	10	11
1:2	1:4	1:8	1:16	1:32	1:64	1:128	1:256	Negative control	Positive control	Patient serum control

████████   LABORATORY WORKSHEET 3

SCHLICTER TEST

Student Name _____

Date performed: _____
Date completed: _____

Predose sample: SIT: _____
Predose sample: SBT: _____

Postdose: SIT: _____
Postdose: SBD: _____

Bibliography

Finegold S M, Baron E: Bailey and Scott's Diagnostic Microbiology, 8th ed. St. Louis: C. V. Mosby Company, 1993.

Howard B, Klaas J, Rubin SJ, Weissfeld A, Tilton R: Clinical and Pathogenic Microbiology, 2nd ed. St. Louis: C. V. Mosby Company, 1994.

Koneman E, Allen SD, Dowell VR, Janda WM, Sommers HM, Winn WC: Color Atlas and Textbook of Diagnostic Microbiology, 4th ed. Philadelphia: J B Lippincott Co, 1990.

Lennette E, Balows A: Manual of Clinical Microbiology, 5th ed. Washington DC: American Society for Microbiology, 1991.

Sherris John: Medical Microbiology: An Introduction to Infectious Diseases, 2nd ed. New York: Elsevier, 1990.

Selected Bacteriologic Culture Media, Stains, and Reagents

Patricia K. Hargrave
Shirley Adams

50. Nutrient Agar
51. Oxidative-Fermentative Medium (Hugh and Leifson Formulation)
52. Peptone-Yeast Extract-Glucose Broth (PYG)
53. Phenylalanine Deaminase Agar (PAD)
54. Phenylethyl Alcohol Agar (PEA)
55. Pseudocel (Cetrimide) Agar
56. Salmonella-Shigella Agar (SS)
57. Selenite F Broth
58. Sodium Chloride Broth, 6.5%
59. SP-4 Broth/Agar
60. SP-4—Arginine, Glucose, and Urea Broths
61. Tetrathionate Broth

62. Thayer-Martin, Modified Agar
63. Thioglycolate Broth
    a. Basal
    b. Enriched
64. Thiosulfate Citrate Bile Salts Sucrose Agar (TCBS)
65. Tinsdale Agar
66. Triple Sugar Iron Agar (TSI)
67. Trypticase Soy Agar (TSA)
68. Trypticase Soy Broth (TSB)
69. Tryptophan Broth (1%)
70. Urea Agar/Broth
71. Vaginalis Agar (V Agar)
72. Xylose-Lysine-Deoxycholate Agar (XLD)

A wide variety of basal, enrichment, selective, and differential media are available to the clinical microbiology laboratory. Each of these media is intended to aid the laboratory in the isolation, cultivation, and identification of clinically significant organisms from patient specimens. A laboratory's efficient performance of these functions is not dependent on its maintaining a vast array of media for routine use. Rather, it is dependent on the laboratory's ability to make wise choices when selecting a routine media menu. Choices should be dictated by factors as discussed in Chapter 7. This appendix is included to provide the reader with more detailed information about a select number of bacteriologic media cited in the bacteriology section of this text. Most of the media detailed in this appendix are commercially available in either dehydrated or finished form.

Preparation of finished media should follow the established formulation and directions. Accuracy in the performance of all weights and measures is essential. All glassware should be chemically clean, and only deionized or distilled water should be used unless the directions specify otherwise. Media rehydrated from powdered formulations should be monitored for appropriate appearance and pH. Media containing agar should be heated to boiling and allowed to boil for approximately 1 minute before sterilizing. Heating and short-term boiling ensure that the agar dissolves completely and guard against charring of the agar during sterilization. Sterilization should be in accord with the formulation's stated directions. Sterility and performance tests (quality controls) should be performed as discussed in Chapter 7.

A7 Agar

A7 agar is a selective-differential medium useful in the isolation of genital mycoplasmas. Although a variety of formulations are available, commonly used formulations contain either penicillin G or penicillin G with amphotericin B to inhibit normal bacterial flora of the genital tract (selective), whereas the presence of horse serum and yeast extract makes it complex enough to support the growth of mycoplasma strains. The addition of urea and manganous sulfate enhances this medium's ability to differentiate *Ureaplasma urealyticum* from mycoplasma strains that do not hydrolyze urea. *U. urealyticum* degradation of urea leads to the production of ammonia. The ammonia produced reacts with manganous sulfate to yield a dark brown product; thus, *U. urealyticum* colonies take on a dark golden brown to deep velvet brown color. *U. urealyticum* colony coloration is in sharp contrast to the clear, light background of the medium. Classic *Mycoplasma*, *Acholeplasma* species, and *Proteus* L colonies do not react to form the colored end product, and colonies remain clear.

Formulation and Preparation

Step 1: Basal Medium. Mix together the following ingredients, adjust the pH to 5.5, and sterilize by autoclaving (121°C for 15 minutes).

Ureaplasma A7 medium, dehydrated	6.6 g
Distilled/deionized water	165 mL

Step 2: Complete Medium. Cool the basal medium to 50°C and add the sterile ingredients listed, mixing well. Adjust to pH 6.2, and dispense into sterile Petri dishes. Allow medium to solidify at room temperature.

Horse serum, unheated	40.0 mL
A commercial enrichment such as:	
Isovitalex (BBL) or GCHI (REMEL)	2.1 mL
Yeast extract, pH 6.0	2.0 mL
Urea, 50%	0.4 mL
L-Cysteine HCl, 4%	0.5 mL
Penicillin, 100,000 units/mL	2.0 mL

Plated complete A7 medium can be stored at 4°C for up to 1 week. *Note:* Although the complete medium can be stored in the refrigerator, the basal medium alone should not be stored. Any plated medium in which a precipitate is observable under the low-power objective of the light microscope should be discarded. Usable, plated medium should be inoculated, streaked for isolation, and incubated anaerobically at 35°C for 48 hours.

Acetate Agar

Acetate agar is a differential medium used to distinguish *Escherichia coli* from *Shigella* species by monitoring the ability to use acetate as the only available carbon source. Organisms capable of using acetate also use the medium's ammonium salt as a nitrogen source. The breakdown of the ammonium salt results in a shift of the pH into the alkaline range. The incorporated pH indicator, bromthymol blue, at alkaline pH shifts in color from green to blue.

Formulation and Preparation

Sodium acetate	2.0	g
Sodium chloride	5.0	g
Monoammonium phosphate	1.0	g
Dipotassium phosphate	1.0	g

Magnesium sulfate	0.2 g
Bromthymol blue	0.08 g
Agar	20.0 g
Distilled/deionized water	1 L

Dissolve dry ingredients in the distilled/deionized water or rehydrate commercial medium according to manufacturer's directions and heat to boiling for 1 minute. Dispense into culture tubes of a size sufficient to accommodate a 3.8-cm slant with a 2.5-cm slant, cap, and sterilize by autoclaving (121°C for 15 minutes). Cool in a slanted position. Final pH of the sterile medium is 6.8. Finished medium should be inoculated by making a saline suspension of a young colony from an agar culture and introducing the saline-suspended organisms onto the slant with a needle. Incubate at 37°C for up to 4 days, while monitoring daily for the expected color change.

Alkaline Peptone Water

Alkaline peptone water is an enrichment medium useful in the recovery of *Vibrio* and *Aeromonas* species from stool specimens. The alkaline pH of this medium allows uninhibited replication of these species while temporarily suppressing the replication rate of many commensal intestinal bacteria.

Formulation and Preparation

Peptone	10.0 g
Sodium chloride	5.0 g
Distilled/deionized water	1 L

Dissolve ingredients in distilled/deionized water, and adjust pH to either 8.6 or 9.0. Some formulations recommend adjusting to pH 9.0 specifically for recovery of vibrios. Disperse into tubes, and sterilize by autoclaving (121°C for 20 minutes). Alkaline peptone water cultures should be incubated at 35°C and subcultured to TCBS agar within 12 to 18 hours.

Bacteroides Bile-Esculin Agar (BBE)

Bacteroides bile-esculin agar is a selective-differential agar used for the isolation and identification of *Bacteroides fragilis*. The incorporation of oxgall (bile salts) separates bile-resistant from bile-sensitive species, whereas the 1% esculin, in conjunction with ferric ammonium, provides information about the isolate's ability to hydrolyze esculin. Products of esculin hydrolysis reacting with the ferric ammonium citrate form an insoluble iron salt that is deposited with the positive colonies, causing them to turn black.

Formulation and Preparation

Trypticase soy agar	40.0 g
Oxgall	20.0 g

Esculin	1.0 g
Ferric ammonium citrate	0.5 g
Hemin solution (5 mg/mL)	2.0 mL
Gentamicin solution (40 mg/mL)	2.5 mL
Distilled/deionized water	1 L

Step 1: Hemin Stock Solution. Hemin stock solution is prepared by dissolving 0.5 g of hemin in 10 mL of 1 N sodium hydroxide, bringing the total volume to 100 mL with distilled/deionized water, and sterilizing by autoclaving (121°C for 15 minutes). Final concentration of the stock solution is 5 mg/mL.

Step 2: Complete Medium. Combine all ingredients and adjust to pH 7.0. Heat to dissolve, and sterilize by autoclaving (121°C for 15 minutes). After autoclaving, cool to 50°C and pour into sterile Petri plates. Plated medium should be inoculated, streaked for isolation, and incubated anaerobically.

Bile Esculin Agar

Bile esculin agar is a selective-differential agar used to isolate and identify group D streptococci, including the enterococci. Oxgall (bile salts) is the selective ingredient, whereas esculin is the differential component. All group D streptococci, including all enterococci, hydrolyze esculin. Products of esculin hydrolysis react with ferric citrate in the medium to produce insoluble iron salts. Deposition of the iron salts results in a blackening of the tubed medium. Test results must be interpreted in conjunction with Gram stain morphology because *Listeria monocytogenes* and a small number of other organisms also react positively.

Formulation and Preparation

Beef extract	3.0 g
Peptone	5.0 g
Oxgall	40.0 g
Esculin	1.0 g
Ferric citrate	0.5 g
Agar	15.0 g
Distilled/deionized water	1 L

Rehydrate commercially available dehydrated medium according to manufacturer's directions. Heat to boiling until dissolved, dispense into screw-cap tubes, and sterilize by autoclaving (121°C for 15 minutes). Cool in slanted position.

Optional Serum Enriched Formulation. Rehydrate commercially available dehydrated medium according to manufacturer's directions. Heat to dissolve, and sterilize by autoclaving. After autoclaving, cool to 55°C and aseptically add 50 mL of sterile horse serum, mixing well. Dispense into sterile screw-cap tubes and allow to finish cooling in a slanted position. Slanted medium should be inoculated, incubated aerobically at 35°C, and observed for growth, with darkening of the medium indicative of esculin hydrolysis.

Bismuth Sulfite Agar

Bismuth sulfite agar is a selective medium for the isolation of *Salmonella* species. The selective ingredients are bismuth sulfite and brilliant green, which inhibit the growth of gram-positive bacteria, most lactose-fermenting intestinal normal flora, and *Shigella* species. Although not a differential medium in the strictest sense, the ferrous sulfate in this medium is reactive with H_2S to produce ferric sulfide, which is deposited within the bacterial colony as a black, insoluble precipitate. Typically, *Salmonella typhi* colonies are black surrounded by a metallic sheen, whereas *Salmonella gallinarum, Salmonella choleraesuis,* and *Salmonella paratyphi* colonies are light green on this medium. When used to isolate *Salmonella* species from feces and other clinical specimens, the parallel use of a less inhibitory medium is recommended because bismuth sulfate agar may inhibit or partially inhibit the growth of some *Salmonella* strains.

Formulation and Preparation

Beef extract	5.0 g
Pancreatic hydrolysate of gelatin, *USP*	10.0 g
Glucose	5.0 g
Disodium phosphate	4.0 g
Ferrous sulfate	0.3 g
Bismuth sulfate	8.0 g
Brilliant green	25 mg
Agar	20.0 g
Distilled/deionized water	1 L

Mix the ingredients or rehydrate the commercially dehydrated medium according to the manufacturer's directions, final pH 7.7. Heat to boiling, cool to 50°C, and dispense as 20-mL aliquots into sterile Petri dishes. To minimize moisture collection on the medium surface, Petri dish lids should be left ajar while the agar solidifies. This medium cannot be autoclaved and must be used on the day it is prepared. Plated medium should be inoculated with fecal or enrichment broth materials, streaked for isolation, and incubated at 35°C for 48 hours.

Blood Agar—Anaerobic, CDC Formulation

CDC anaerobic blood agar is an enrichment medium useful in the isolation and culture of fastidious anaerobes.

Formulation and Preparation

Trypticase soy agar	40.0 g
Agar	5.0 g
Yeast extract	5.0 g
L-Cysteine	0.4 g
Hemin	5 mg

Vitamin K₁ stock solution   1 mL
Distilled/deionized water   950 mL

Step 1: Solutions. Prepare fresh hemin–L-cysteine solution by dissolving 500 mg of hemin and 400 mg of L-cystene in 5 mL of 1 N sodium hydroxide. This solution should not be stored for later use.

Prepare vitamin K₁ stock solution by adding 1 g of vitamin K₁ in 99 mL of absolute ethanol. Prepared solution may be stored in a sterile brown bottle at 4°C.

Step 2: Complete Medium. Mix all ingredients and heat to dissolve. Adjust to final pH 7.4 and sterilize by autoclaving (121°C for 15 minutes). After autoclaving, cool to 50°C, and add 50 mL of sterile defibrinated sheep blood. Agitate gently to mix, and dispense into sterile Petri dishes. Plated medium can be stored for up to 6 weeks if sealed in cellophane bags and stored at 4°C. Usable plates should be inoculated, streaked for isolation, and incubated anaerobically at 35°C for 48 hours.

Blood Agar—Anaerobic, Brucella Base (Wadsworth)

Brucella base anaerobic blood agar is a useful enrichment medium for the isolation of moderately fastidious, obligate anaerobes. Sheep blood provides the enrichment.

Formulation and Preparation

Pancreatic digest of casein	10.0 g
Peptic digest of animal tissues	10.0 g
Glucose	1.0 g
Yeast extract	2.0 g
Sodium chloride	5.0 g
Sodium bisulfate	0.1 g
Agar	15.0 g
Hemin (5 mg/mL)	1.0 mL
Vitamin K₁ (10 mg/mL)	1.0 mL
Distilled/deionized water	950 mL

Step 1: Stock Solutions. Prepare the hemin solution by dissolving 500 mg of hemin in 5 mL of 1 N sodium hydroxide. Prepare vitamin K₁ solution as for CDC anaerobic blood agar.

Step 2: Basal Medium. Rehydrate commercially available dehydrated Brucella agar according to manufacturer's directions, final pH 7.0. Add 1 mL of hemin solution, mix, and sterilize by autoclaving (121°C for 15 minutes).

Step 3: Complete Medium. Cool sterile basal medium to 55°C; aseptically add 1 mL of vitamin K₁ solution and 50 mL of sterile defibrinated sheep blood. Agitate gently to mix and dispense into sterile Petri plates. Plated medium should be sealed in bags and stored at 4°C for up to 2 weeks. Usable plates are inoculated, streaked for isolation, and incubated anaerobically at 35°C for 48 hours.

Blood Agar—Anaerobic, with Kanamycin and Vancomycin (KV Blood Agar)

KV blood agar is a variation of CDC anaerobic blood agar made semiselective by the addition of antibiotics. It is useful in the primary isolation of obligate anaerobes, particularly *Bacteroides* species, from specimens with a mixed bacterial population.

Formulation and Preparation

Step 1: Stock Antibiotic Solutions. To prepare the kanamycin stock solution, dissolve 1 g of kanamycin (base activity) in 10 mL of sterile, pH 8.0 phosphate buffer. Stock solution kanamycin concentration is 100,000 μg/mL. The stock solution can be stored at 4°C for up to 1 year and is autoclavable.

To prepare the vancomycin stock solution, dissolve 75 mg of vancomycin (base activity) in 5 mL of 0.05 N HCl and add 5 mL of sterile distilled water. Stock solution vancomycin concentration is 7,500 μg/mL. The stock solution can be stored for up to 1 month at 4°C or up to 1 year at −20°C. This stock solution cannot be autoclaved.

Step 2: Complete Medium. Prepare CDC anaerobic blood agar. After adding the sheep blood, aseptically add 1 mL of kanamycin stock solution (100 mg base activity) and 1 mL of vancomycin (7.5 mg base activity). Dispense complete medium into Petri dishes. Plated medium can be placed in bags and the bags sealed and stored at 4°C for up to 4 weeks. Usable plates should be inoculated, streaked for isolation, and incubated anaerobically at 35°C for 48 hours. Plates negative at 48 hours may be reincubated, depending on the particular situation.

Blood Agar—Anaerobic, Laked with Kanamycin and Vancomycin (KVKL)

Anaerobic, laked blood agar with kanamycin, vancomycin, and vitamin K_1 (KVKL) is an enrichment-selective medium recommended for the isolation of species of *Bacteroides* and *Prevotella* from clinical specimens. Although appropriate for the isolation of any *Bacteroides* species, this medium is particularly helpful in the isolation of *Prevotella melaninogenica* because pigment production is enhanced. Lake erythrocytes and vitamin K_1 constitute the enrichment ingredients, whereas the antibiotics inhibit all cocci and facultative gram-negative bacilli except the pseudomonads.

Formulation and Preparation

Pancreatic digest of casein/peptic digest of animal tissue	20.0 g
Glucose	1.0 g
Yeast extract	2.0 g
Sodium chloride	5.0 g
Sodium bisulfate	0.1 g
Agar	15.0 g

Hemin (5 mg/mL)	1.0 mL
Vitamin K_1 (10 mg/mL)	1.0 mL
Kanamycin (100 mg/mL)	1.0 mL
Vancomycin (7.5 mg/mL)	1.0 mL
Laked sheep blood	50.0 mL
Distilled/deionized water	950 mL

Step 1: Enrichment and Antibiotic Solutions. Prepare hemin solution as for Brucella anaerobic blood agar. Prepare vitamin K_1 solution as for CDC anaerobic blood agar. Prepare kanamycin and vancomycin stock solutions as for KV blood agar. Prepare laked sheep blood by freezing whole blood overnight and thawing before use.

Step 2: Basal Medium. The basal medium is commercially available in dehydrated form as Brucella agar. Rehydrate commercial medium according to manufacturer's directions, final pH 7.0. Add the hemin, vitamin K_1, and kanamycin solution; heat to dissolve, and sterilize by autoclaving (121°C for 15 minutes).

Step 3: Complete Medium. Cool sterile basal medium to 50°C; aseptically add 1 mL of vancomycin and 50 mL of laked sheep blood; dispense into sterile Petri dishes. Plated medium should be inoculated, streaked for isolation, and incubated anaerobically at 35°C for a minimum of 48 hours.

Blood Agar, Sheep (SBA)

Blood agar is a routine enrichment medium used to cultivate a wide variety of moderately fastidious bacterial organisms. An infusion agar or tryptic soy agar base can be enriched by the addition of 5 to 10% defibrinated sheep, rabbit, or human blood. Sheep blood, however, has proved the most versatile enrichment. Incorporation of the blood not only provides enrichment for growth of the bacterial organisms, but also allows the detection and characterization of hemolytic activity.

Formulation and Preparation

Step 1: Basal Medium.

Pancreatic digest of casein	15.0 g
Soy bean peptone	5.0 g
Sodium chloride	5.0 g
Agar	15.0 g
Distilled/deionized water	950 mL

Rehydrate commercially available dehydrated infusion or trypticase soy agar according to manufacturer's directions, final pH 7.3. Heat to boiling, and sterilize by autoclaving (121°C for 15 minutes).

Step 2: Complete Medium. Cool sterile base medium to 50°C; aseptically add 50 mL of defibrinated sheep blood and mix by gentle agitation using a motion that minimizes the incorporation of air bubbles. Dispense into sterile Petri dishes. If plates are to be prepared by pouring, care should be taken to avoid the incorporation of air bubbles. If air bubbles are present in newly poured medium, quickly pass the flame of a Bunsen burner over the medium surface before it solidifies. This breaks the bubbles. Plated medium should be placed in plastic bags to minimize moisture loss and stored at 4°C. Usable plates should be inoculated, streaked, and incubated as dictated by the specific application.

Blood Agar, Rabbit

Rabbit blood agar is an enrichment medium particularly useful in the recovery and demonstration of β hemolysis by *Haemophilus influenzae* and *Gardnerella vaginalis*.

Formulation and Preparation

Preparation is the same as for sheep blood agar, with defibrinated rabbit blood replacing the sheep blood. Storage and inoculation are the same as for sheep blood agar.

Blood Phenylethyl Alcohol Agar—Anaerobic, CDC Formulation

Phenylethyl alcohol agar (PEA) is an enrichment-selective medium useful in the isolation of *Bacteroides, Prevotella,* and other obligate anaerobes from specimens containing a mixture of obligate and facultative anaerobes. Enrichment is provided by yeast extract, hemin, vitamin K_1, and defibrinated sheep blood. Selectivity is provided by the incorporation of phenylethyl alcohol, which inhibits facultative anaerobes by suppressing DNA synthesis and cell division.

Formulation and Preparation

Pancreatic digest of casein, *USP*	15.0 g
Papaic digest of soybean meal, *USP*	5.0 g
Sodium chloride	5.0 g
Yeast extract	5.0 g
Phenylethyl alcohol	2.5 g
Agar	20.0 g
Distilled/deionized water	1 L

Step 1: Stock Solutions. Prepare hemin, cysteine solution as for CDC anaerobic blood agar. Prepare vitamin K_1 solution as for CDC anaerobic blood agar.

Step 2: Basal Medium. Mix ingredients or rehydrate commercially available dehydrated base agar according to manufacturer's directions, heat to boiling, and add the hemin–L-cysteine and vitamin K_1 solutions. Sterilize by autoclaving (121°C for 15 minutes).

Step 3: Complete Medium. Cool the sterile basal medium to 50°C and aseptically add sterile defibrinated sheep blood, agitating gently to mix. Dispense into sterile Petri dishes. Plated medium should be sealed in plastic bags for storage. Bagged plates may be stored up to 4 weeks at 4°C. Usable plates should be inoculated, streaked for isolation, and incubated anaerobically at 35°C for at least 48 hours.

Blood Phenylethyl Alcohol Agar, Wadsworth

Wadsworth blood phenylethyl alcohol agar is an alternative to the CDC formulation of blood phenylethyl alcohol agar. Similar to the CDC formulation, it is a selective medium for the isolation of *Bacteroides* and *Prevotella* species. The inoculation, incubation, and interpretation of growth on this medium are the same as for the CDC blood phenylethyl alcohol agar discussed previously.

Formulation and Preparation

Step 1: Basal Medium.

Phenylethyl alcohol agar	42.5 g
Vitamin K_1 (10 mg/mL)	1.0 mL
Distilled/deionized water	949 mL

Rehydrate commercial agar in the distilled/deionized water according to manufacturer's instructions and add vitamin K_1. Bring to boiling, and sterilize by autoclaving (121°C for 15 minutes).

Step 2: Complete Medium. Cool the sterile basal medium to 50°C; add 50 mL of sterile, defibrinated sheep blood; and agitate gently to produce a uniform suspension. Dispense into Petri plates. Usable plated medium can be stored bagged for 2 weeks at 4°C.

Bordet-Gengou Blood Agar (B-G)

Bordet-Gengou blood agar is an enrichment-selective medium for the isolation of *Bordetella pertussis* and *Bordetella parapertussis* from clinical specimens. Formulations for the base medium vary with respect to the use of peptone. Growth on the peptone-free formulation is less luxuriant, and indigenous flora is less likely to overgrow the pathogen; hence the formulation without peptone should be used for isolation by the "cough plate" method. The base medium formulation with peptone is suitable for isolation if a nasopharyngeal swab specimen is obtained. The complete medium is enriched by the addition of glycerol and sterile, defibrinated sheep blood. Increased selectivity of the complete medium has been achieved historically by adding penicillin, methicillin, or cephalexin to the medium just before plating.

Formulation and Preparation

Step 1: Basal Medium.

Potato infusion	125.0 g
Peptone*	10.0 g

Sodium chloride   5.5 g
Agar   20.0 g

Rehydrate dehydrated medium according to manufacturer's directions. Heat to boiling for 1 minute, dispense 20-mL volumes into screw-cap tubes, and sterilize by autoclaving (121°C for 15 minutes). Tubed basal medium may be stored at 4°C for up to 1 year. Stored basal medium should be melted to prepare plates as needed.

Step 2: Complete Medium. Liquid basal medium should be cooled to approximately 50°C before adding the blood and antibiotic. In formulations using selective antibiotic (penicillin at 0.25 to 0.5 units/mL finished medium, 65 μL of a 100 μg/mL methicillin stock solution, or 5 to 40 μg/mL cephalexin), the antibiotic should be added aseptically just before the addition of the blood enrichment. Blood enrichment between 15 and 30% (3 to 6 mL/20 mL tube) is appropriate and determined by the preference of the laboratory. The species from which the sterile, defibrinated blood is obtained is not critical, but properly prepared plates should be cherry-red, moist, and bubble free. Complete, plated medium should be used immediately if possible. If for some reason this is not possible, plates, if tightly sealed, can be maintained for about 1 week at 4°C. Usable, complete medium can be inoculated as a cough plate or by rolling the nasopharyngeal swab specimen over one third of the plate surface and streaking for isolation with a platinum loop. The specimen should be inoculated in this fashion onto B-G plates without antibiotic and B-G plates with antibiotic. Inoculated plates should be incubated at 35 to 37°C for examination at 48 hours. Plates negative at 48 hours should be reincubated. Plates must be held 5 days before regarding as negative for the organism.

Brain-Heart Infusion Broth

Brain-heart infusion broth is an enriched medium suitable for the cultivation of a number of nonfastidious and moderately fastidious microorganisms. This broth medium is recommended for cultivation of pneumococci for the bile solubility test.

Formulation and Preparation

Calf brain infusion	200.0 g
Beef heart infusion	250.0 g
Proteose or gelysate peptone	10.0 g
Dextrose	2.0 g
Sodium chloride	5.0 g
Disodium phosphate	2.5 g
Distilled/deionized water	1 L

Rehydrate powdered medium according to manufacturer's directions, and verify final pH 7.4. Dispense desired volume into culture tubes, cap, and sterilize by autoclaving (121°C for 15 minutes).

Buffered Charcoal-Yeast Extract Agar with α-Ketoglutarate (BCYE-α)

Buffered charcoal-yeast extract agar with α-ketoglutarate is an enrichment medium useful in the isolation of *Legionella* species from clinical specimens. Yeast extract and L-cysteine enhance the growth of *Legionella* organisms, while activated charcoal absorbs toxic compounds that either accumulate as a result of organismal metabolism or are present following preparation of this medium.

Formulation and Preparation

Step 1: Basal Medium.

ACES (N-2-acetamido-2-ethanesulfonic acid)	10.0 g
Monopotassium α-ketoglutarate	1.0 g
Agar	17.0 g
Yeast extract	10.0 g
Activated charcoal (Norit SG-acid and alkali washed)	2.0 g
Distilled/deionized water	930 mL

Add ACES and α-ketoglutarate to water at room temperature and adjust pH with 1 N potassium hydroxide. *Note:* Different laboratories adjust to different pHs at this point to obtain a solid medium with a final pH of 6.9. CDC recommends adjusting the pH at this point to 7.2, whereas others recommend 6.9. Adjustments must be made with potassium hydroxide rather than sodium hydroxide because sodium hydroxide might lead to an inhibitory effect. After adjustment of the pH, add agar, dissolve by boiling, and add yeast extract with charcoal. Mix and sterilize by autoclaving (121°C for 15 minutes).

Step 2: Additive Solutions. Prepare L-cysteine solution by dissolving 0.4 g of L-cysteine hydrochloride in 10 mL of distilled/deionized water and filter sterilizing. Prepare ferric pyrophosphate by dissolving 0.25 g of ferric pyrophosphate crystals in 10 mL of distilled/deionized water and filter sterilizing. Both solutions must be made fresh at the time the medium is made. Ferric pyrophosphate crystals to be used for solution preparation must be kept dry and should be discarded if crystal color changes from chartreuse to brown.

Step 3: Complete Medium. Cool sterile basal medium to 50°C; add the L-cysteine (10 mL) and ferric pyrophosphate (10 mL) solutions, always adding the L-cysteine first. Dispense medium, in approximately 20-mL volumes to minimize drying, into sterile Petri dishes. Gentle agitation during the dispensing process is necessary to keep the charcoal uniformly suspended. One plate from every batch of this medium should be used to verify a final pH of 6.85 − 6.95. Usable plated medium may be stored in plastic bags, away from light, at 4°C for up to 4 weeks. Plated medium should be inoculated, streaked for isolation, and incubated at 35°C in a CO_2 incubator. Cultures should be checked daily for up to 2 weeks and incubator humidity monitored to prevent excessive drying of plates. *Legionella* colonies may not be grossly visible until 3 to 5 days after inoculation.

BCYE-α, L-Cysteine Deficient

This medium is a variation of buffered charcoal-yeast extract agar with α-ketoglutarate (BCYE-α). Its formulation is identical with the exception of L-

cysteine. This medium, deficient in L-cysteine, is helpful in presumptively sepa-
rating those gram-negative, non-*Legionella* organisms that may grow on BCYE-
α from *Legionella* species. Non-*Legionella* gram-negative rods grow in the
absence of L-cysteine, whereas *Legionella* species do not. Consequently, growth
on both cysteine-containing and cysteine-deficient medium suggests the isolate
is not a *Legionella* species, whereas growth on the cysteine-containing medium
suggests only a requirement for L-cysteine that is characteristic of *Legionella*
species. Preparation, storage, and use are identical to that of BCYE-α.

BCYE-α, With Antibiotics

This is a semiselective variation of BCYE-α useful in the isolation of *Legionella* species from body sites that contain a mixed bacterial flora. Three antibiotics are added to the standard BCYE-α formulation to inhibit the growth of other
bacteria and fungi. Cefamandole inhibits gram-positive organisms, polymyxin
B inhibits gram-negative bacilli, especially pseudomonads, and anisomycin
inhibits fungi.

BCYE-α, Modified Wadowsky-Yee (mWY)

This is also a semiselective variation of BCYE-α useful in the isolation of
Legionella species from body sites that contain a mixed bacterial flora. This
variation uses glycine and polymyxin B to inhibit gram-negative organisms,
vancomycin to inhibit gram-positive cocci, and anisomycin to inhibit fungi.

Formulation and Preparation

Step 1: BCYE-α. Prepare standard BCYE-α formulation plus 3 g of glycine.
Step 2: Additive Solutions. Prepare and filter sterilize the following solutions: 10 mg of bromcresol purple in a small volume of 0.1 N KOH; 10 mg of
bromthymol blue in a small volume of 0.1 N KOH; a combined antibiotic solution
containing 1 mL vancomycin, 50,000 units of polymyxin B sulfate, and 80 mg of
anisomycin in 10 mL of distilled water.
Step 3: Complete Medium. Aseptically add filter sterilized, additive solutions to BCYE-α with glycine and dispense into sterile Petri dishes. Store and
use in the same fashion as BCYE-α and BCYE-α with antibiotics.

Campylobacter Blood Agar (CAMPY-BA)

Campylobacter blood agar is an enrichment-selective medium useful in
the isolation and cultivation of *Campylobacter* species from stool specimens.
Brucella agar serves as the base medium for CAMPY-BA because it contains
sodium bisulfate, which lowers the redox potential, thereby enhancing the
recovery of microaerophilic organisms such as *Campylobacter* species. Ten
percent sheep blood enriches the basal medium, and an antibiotic cocktail
makes the medium selective. Although minor variations exist in the composition

of this cocktail, most formulations have incorporated vancomycin to inhibit the gram-positive cocci, trimethoprim to inhibit swarming strains of *Proteus,* polymyxin B to inhibit the gram-negative bacilli, and amphotericin B to inhibit the filamentous fungi and yeasts. Currently, cefoperazone is being promoted to replace cephalothin. Cefoperazone has antipseudomonal activity (lacked by cephalothin) and is more effective against members of the *Enterobacteriaceae.*

Formulation and Preparation

Step 1: Basal Medium. Prepare commercially available dehydrated Brucella agar in 900 mL of distilled/deionized water according to manufacturer's directions, and sterilize by autoclaving (121°C for 15 minutes).

Step 2: Complete Medium. Cool sterile basal medium to 50°C and aseptically add the following ingredients:

Sterile defibrinated sheep blood	100 mL
Vancomycin	10 mg
Trimethroprim	5 mg
Polymyxin B	2,500 IU
Amphotericin B	2 mg
Cephalothin	15 mg

Dispense complete medium into sterile Petri dishes and store at 4°C.

Campylobacter Thioglycolate Broth (CAMPY-Thio)

CAMPY-Thio is a selective liquid medium. The base medium is thioglycolate broth with 0.16% agar. The selective component is the antibiotic cocktail used in CAMPY-BA.

Carbohydrate Fermentation Media, Anaerobic

Carbohydrate broths are differential media useful in determining the ability to ferment specific carbohydrates. This formulation, based on a carbohydrate medium base (Difco), is useful in the determination of carbohydrate fermentations carried out by anaerobic isolates.

Formulation and Preparation

Step 1: Base Medium.

CHO medium base (Difco)	26.0 g
Distilled/deionized water	900.0 mL

Rehydrate commercially available dehydrated medium according to manufacturer's directions, sterilize by autoclaving (121°C for 15 minutes), and cool to 50°C.

Step 2: Test Carbohydrates/Complete Medium. Aqueous carbohydrate stock solutions except for starch are prepared by dissolving 6 g of the carbohydrate in 100 mL of distilled/deionized water (6% solution) and filter sterilizing. The starch stock solution is prepared by dissolving 2.5 g of starch in 100 mL of distilled/deionized water (2.5% solution) and filter sterilizing. Aseptically add the 100 mL of filter sterilized carbohydrate solution to the cooled base medium and adjust the pH to 7.0 + 0.1 at room temperature. Aseptically dispense as 7-mL volumes into sterile 15 × 90 mm screw-capped tubes. Tubed medium may be stored at room or refrigerator temperature, but dissolved oxygen must be removed either before storage or before use. If an anaerobic chamber is available, the tubed medium, loosely capped, should be passed into the anaerobic atmosphere (85% N_2; 10% H_2; 5% CO_2) and the caps securely tightened before removal and storage. If an anaerobic chamber is not available, the tubed medium should be steamed or boiled with the caps loose for 10 minutes, cooled, and inoculated immediately using a capillary pipette to deliver the inoculum near the bottom of the tube without introducing air. One pipette may be used to inoculate multiple tubes. All cultures should be incubated anaerobically, with the caps loosened, at 35°C for up to 7 days. Cultures should be examined on days 1, 2, and 7 for fermentation with production of acid. At pH 6.0 or lower, the bromthymol blue indicator burns yellow, indicating a positive fermentation reaction. If fermentation does not occur, the bromthymol blue indicator remains blue to blue-green (negative reaction). If the cultured organism can reduce the bromthymol indicator, the medium becomes colorless. If this occurs, a sterile pipette can be used to transfer two to three drops of material from the tube(s) involved to a spot plate. Two to three drops of dilute indicator are then added to the transferred material and observed for color change. *Note:* Rapid test systems are available that include carbohydrate fermentations with a bromcresol purple indicator. Correlation between fermentation and color change is similar, as is the problem of indicator reduction and the method for detecting acid in the presence of reduced indicator.

Carbohydrate Fermentation Media, Gram-Positive Cocci

Carbohydrate broths are differential media useful in determining the ability of a variety of aerobic bacteria to ferment specific carbohydrates. This formulation, based on a heart infusion broth, provides sufficient nutrients to support the growth of gram-positive cocci, including the streptococci.

Formulation and Preparation

Step 1: Basal Medium.

Heart muscle infusion	375 g
Thiotone peptone	10 g
Sodium chloride	5 g
Distilled/deionized water	1 L
Bromcresol purple indicator (1.6 g/100 mL 95% ethanol)	1 mL

Rehydrate commercially available dehydrated heart infusion broth according to manufacturer's directions, and add pH indicator (bromcresol purple). *Note:* If the carbohydrate to be incorporated is stable at autoclave temperature and pressure, 10 g of the specific carbohydrate can be added at this time. If the carbohydrate can be autoclaved, all ingredients should be dissolved, dispensed as 3-mL aliquots into screw-cap tubes, and sterilized by autoclaving either at reduced temperature and pressure (116°C to 118°C at 10 to 12 pounds pressure for 15 minutes) or at standard temperature and pressure for a shorter time (121°C for 10 minutes). If the carbohydrate to be incorporated is not stable, dissolve heart infusion broth and indicator, stopper, and autoclave in the flask to sterilize (121°C for 15 minutes).

Step 2: Test Carbohydrate/Complete Medium. Some test carbohydrates useful in the differentiation of gram-positive cocci do not withstand the temperature and pressure associated with autoclaving. In the case of these test carbohydrates, a 5 to 10% solution should be prepared, depending on that carbohydrate's solubility, and filter sterilized. The sterile carbohydrate should be added to the sterile basal medium (cooled to 50°C) to give a 1% final concentration. Tubed carbohydrate fermentation medium should be inoculated and incubated aerobically at 35°C. A positive reaction (acid production) is indicated by a color change from purple to yellow.

Carbohydrate Fermentation Media, Aerobic Gram-Negative Bacilli

A carbohydrate fermentation medium of this formulation does not contain sufficient quantities of complex nutrients to support the growth of fastidious aerobic bacteria. It is, however, sufficient to support the less fastidious *Enterobacteriaceae;* thus, it is the formulation of choice to determine the fermentative patterns of suspect *Enterobacteriaceae* isolates.

Formulation and Preparation

Peptone	10.0 g
Sodium chloride	5.0 g
Andrade indicator	10.0 mL
Test carbohydrate	10.0 g
Distilled/deionized water	1 L

Step 1: Andrade pH Indicator. Prepare Andrade reagent by dissolving 0.5 g of acid fuchsin in 100 mL of distilled/deionized water. When fuchsin is dissolved, add 15 mL of 1 N sodium hydroxide and set aside for several hours. If after several hours this solution has not changed color (from red to brown), add an additional 1 to 2 mL of the 1 N sodium hydroxide, drop by drop, until the solution is straw-yellow in color. This reagent should be stored (aged) for approximately 6 months before use.

Step 2: Basal Medium. Prepare peptone broth base with Andrade indicator, heat to dissolve, and sterilize by autoclaving.

Step 3: Test Carbohydrate/Complete Medium. Test carbohydrates are prepared as for the infusion broth formulation, and the same special conditions must be addressed. If the test carbohydrate does not tolerate autoclaving, the sterile basal medium should be cooled to 50°C and the filter sterilized carbohydrate solution added. Tubed media should be inoculated and incubated aerobically at 35°C. A positive result (acid production) is indicated by a color change from yellow or colorless (alkaline) to pink or red.

Chocolate Agar

Chocolate agar is an enrichment agar especially useful in promoting the growth of *Haemophilus* and other fastidious bacterial species. A variation of sheep blood agar, this medium may be made by adding the sheep blood while the basal medium is warm enough to release the red cell hemoglobin and nicotinamide adenine dinucleotide (NAD). Alternatively the sheep blood may be replaced by 2% hemoglobin and a chemical supplement solution. The enrichment used must result in the complete medium containing cell-free hemoglobin and nicotinamide dinucleotide (NAD). The temperature at which either enrichment is added results in a chocolate-brown colored medium.

Formulation and Preparation

Step 1: Basal Medium.

Pancreatic digest of casein/peptic digest of animal tissue (polypeptone/proteose peptone)	15.0 g
Cornstarch	1.0 g
Sodium chloride	5.0 g
Dipotassium phosphate	4.0 g
Monopotassium phosphate	1.0 g
Agar	10.0 g

Proteose agar and GC agar are commercially available dehydrated agar formulations that can serve as the basal medium for preparation of chocolate agar. Prepare the basal medium double strength by rehydrating the commercially available, dehydrated medium using the normal quantity of powdered material in one half the usual volume of distilled/deionized water, final pH 7.3. Mix, heat to boiling to dissolve, and sterilize by autoclaving (121°C for 15 minutes).

Step 2: Complete Medium. If sheep blood is to be used as the enrichment, cool sterile basal medium to 70°C, aseptically add the sterile defibrinated sheep blood, and heat to 80°C for 15 minutes or until the medium turns brown. If hemin and a chemical enrichment are to be used to complete the medium, aseptically add 2% sterile hemoglobin and a chemical supplement, such as Isovitalex, to basal medium cooled to 70°C. Once the supplement is added, cool the complete medium to 50°C and dispense into sterile Petri dishes. Plated medium can be stored at 4°C. Usable plates should be inoculated, streaked for isolation, and incubated at 35°C in CO_2.

Citrate Agar, Simmons

Simmons citrate agar is useful in differentiating gram-negative enteric bacilli. Similar in principle to acetate agar, citrate replaces acetate in this medium, and differentiation is based on the isolate's ability or inability to use citrate as its sole source of carbon. Several alternate theories have been advanced to explain the biochemical sequences leading to a color change in this medium. One such theory holds that, as with acetate agar, organisms capable of using the citrate also use the medium's ammonium salt as a nitrogen source. The breakdown of the ammonium salt results in a shift of the pH into the alkaline range. The incorporated pH indicator, bromthymol blue, at alkaline pH shifts in color from green to blue.

Formulation and Preparation

Ammonium dihydrogen phosphate	1.0	g
Dipotassium phosphate	1.0	g
Sodium citrate	2.0	g
Sodium chloride	5.0	g
Magnesium sulfate	0.2	g
Bromthymol blue	0.08	g
Agar	15.0	g
Distilled/deionized water	1	L

Rehydrate commercial medium according to manufacturer's directions, and heat to boiling for 1 minute. Disperse into culture tubes of a size sufficient to accommodate a 3.8-cm slant with a 2.5-cm slant, cap, and sterilize by autoclaving (121°C for 15 minutes). Cool in a slanted position. Final pH of the sterile medium is 6.9±. Finished medium should be inoculated by making a saline suspension of a young colony from an agar culture, streaking the saline-suspended organisms onto the slant with a needle and stabbing the butt. Inoculated slants should be incubated at 35°C for up to 4 days and monitored daily for the expected color change.

Columbia Agar Base Without Antibiotics

Columbia agar is a basal nutrient agar that contains peptones derived from both casein and meat. The basal medium is suitable for cultivation of a number of aerobic and anaerobic bacterial organisms found in clinical materials. Additionally, it provides an efficient base for preparation of a variety of enrichment agars that support the growth of more fastidious aerobes and anaerobes.

Formulation and Preparation

Step 1: Basal Medium.

Pancreatic digest of casein/peptic digest of animal tissue (polypeptone peptone)	10.0 g
Pancreatic digest of casein with yeast autolysate (biosate peptone)	10.0 g
Pancreatic digest of heart muscle (myosate peptone)	3.0 g
Cornstarch	1.0 g
Sodium chloride	5.0 g

Agar	13.5 g
Distilled/deionized water	1 L

Rehydrate commercially available dehydrated medium according to manufacturer's directions. Dissolve by heating and sterilize by autoclaving (121°C for 15 minutes).

Step 2: Complete Medium. Cool sterile basal medium to temperature appropriate for addition of specific enrichment ingredients necessary to produce final enrichment or enrichment-selective medium. Pour into sterile Petri plates, cool, and store as appropriate for the specific complete medium made. Inoculate plated medium, streak for isolation, and incubate at 35°C for up to 7 days as appropriate for the specific organism to be cultured.

Columbia Agar With Antibiotics (Columbia CNA)

Columbia agar with antibiotics is an enrichment-selective medium suitable for the isolation of gram-positive cocci from specimens that might also be expected to contain gram-negative bacilli, especially *Proteus* species. Sheep blood is the usual enrichment ingredient, whereas colistin and nalidixic acid are incorporated to inhibit gram-negative overgrowth of desired gram-positive isolates.

Formulation and Preparation

Step 1: Basal Medium.

Pancreatic digest of casein/peptic digest of animal tissue (polypeptone peptone)	10.0 g
Pancreatic digest of casein with yeast autolysate (biosate peptone)	10.0 g
Pancreatic digest of heart muscle (myosate peptone)	3.0 g
Cornstarch	1.0 g
Sodium chloride	5.0 g
Agar	13.5 g
Colistin	10.0 mg
Nalidixic acid	15.0 mg
Distilled/deionized water	1 L

Rehydrate commercially available dehydrated medium according to manufacturer's directions. Dissolve by heating, and sterilize by autoclaving (121°C for 15 minutes).

Step 2: Complete Medium. Cool sterile base medium to 50°C; aseptically add 5% defibrinated sterile sheep blood and any other additives appropriate to recovery of the specific suspect bacterial species; dispense into sterile Petri plates. Plated medium should be inoculated, streaked for isolation, and incubated in an environment appropriate to the isolation of the desired species.

Cooked Meat Medium

Cooked meat medium is useful in the cultivation of anaerobes, especially pathogenic species of *Clostridium*. This medium contains solid meat particles and is excellent for initiating growth from a small inoculum as well as sustaining culture viability over long periods. It is useful for cultivation of mixed cultures because all organisms are supported, whereas overgrowth by the more rapid growers is retarded.

Formulation and Preparation

Beef heart	454.0 g
Pancreatic digest of casein and peptic digest of animal tissue (polypeptone or proteose peptone)	20.0 g
Dextrose	2.0 g
Sodium chloride	5.0 g
Distilled/deionized water	1 L
Final pH 7.2 ± 0.2	

Suspend dehydrated medium in tubes according to manufacturer's directions. Allow tubed materials to stand until thoroughly moistened (approximately 15 minutes) before sterilizing by autoclaving (121°C for 15 minutes). Tubed medium may be stored at room temperature, but stored tubes should be placed in flowing steam or a boiling water bath for 10 minutes to drive off dissolved gases and cooled rapidly before inoculating. Cooled, tubed medium should be inoculated and incubated in a manner appropriate for the species being isolated or subcultured. Proteolytic activity by cultured organisms is usually evidenced by blackening of the medium with digestion of the meat particles. Saccharolytic clostridial species typically produce acid with gas. *Note:* A variation of this medium, cooked meat phytone medium, adds calcium carbonate particles and phytone (1.5%) to the original formulation. Cooked meat phytone supports the growth of pathogenic and butyric-butyl clostridial species as well as fusiforms, bacteroides, and other anaerobic non–spore-formers. If subcultures are of strict anaerobes or specimens are suspected to contain strict anaerobes of interest, growth may be expedited by anaerobic incubation. Proteolytic activity by the cultured organism(s) is evidenced by digestion of the meat particles, possibly with darkening of the medium.

Tellurite Blood Agar (With/Without Cystine)

Tellurite blood agar is an enrichment-selective differential agar useful in the isolation of *Corynebacterium diphtheriae*. All formulations include animal blood as a source of enrichment. Some formulations (Frobisher) also incorporate cystine to enhance further the growth of fastidious organisms including *C. diphtheriae*. Potassium tellurite is the selective differential ingredient responsible for inhibiting the growth of staphylococci and streptococci while allowing the growth of *C. diphtheriae* and diphtheroids that act on the tellurite depositing the reduced product within the colonies.

Formulation and Preparation

Step 1: Basal Medium. Either infusion agar or dextrose proteose no. 3 agar is a suitable base for the complete medium. Both are available commercially in dehydrated form. Either should be rehydrated according to the manufacturer's instructions, heated to boiling before dispensing as 15-mL volumes into screw-capped tubes, and sterilized by autoclaving (121°C for 15 minutes). Tubes of base medium may be stored and melted to make the complete medium as culture plates are needed.

Step 2: Complete Medium. If the *Frobisher formulation* is being made, a tube of infusion agar is melted and cooled to and maintained at 50°C while the following ingredients are aseptically added: (1) Cystine (0.45 to 0.75 mg/15 mL of medium) is added as a dry powder, which does not require sterilization; (2) 2.25 mL of a 0.3% aqueous potassium tellurite solution previously sterilized by filtration or autoclaving is added; (3) 1.0 mL of sterile defibrinated blood is added. If the *Kellogg-Wende formulation* is being made, a tube of the base dextrose proteose no. 3 agar is melted and cooled to and maintained at 75°C while aseptically adding 0.75 mL of 0.8% sterile aqueous potassium tellurite and 1.0 mL of sterile defibrinated rabbit blood. Tubes are then cooled to 45 to 50°C before pouring into sterile Petri dishes. Freshly plated medium should be inoculated, streaked for isolation, and incubated at 35°C. On this medium, colonies of *C. diphtheriae* are dull gray-black, whereas diphtheroids are light gray-green with dark centers. Some *Staphylococcus* species, gram-negative bacilli, and yeasts may overcome inhibition and grow on this medium. The *Staphylococcus* colonies are large, glistening, and jet-black, whereas those of the gram-negative bacilli and yeast are dull gray-black but larger than the *C. diphtheriae* colonies.

Cystine Tryptophan Agar With Sugar (CTA-Sugars)

Cystine tryptophan (tryptic/trypticase) agar is a semisolid base medium that contains no meat or plant extracts and is free of fermentable carbohydrates. It may be made differential by the addition of a carbohydrate (CTA-sugar). CTA-sugars are recommended for the determination of fermentation reactions by fastidious organisms.

Formulation and Preparation

Step 1: Basal Medium.

Pancreatic digest of casein (tryptose/trypticase)	20.0 g
Cystine	0.5 g
Sodium chloride	5.0 g
Sodium sulfite	0.5 g
Agar	2.5 g
Phenol red	17 mg
Distilled/deionized water	1 L
Final pH 7.3 ± 0.2	

Rehydrate commercially available dehydrated medium according to manufacturer's instructions, and heat until ingredients are thoroughly dissolved and sterilized by autoclaving. If sugars are incorporated before autoclaving, the tubed medium should be autoclaved at 115 to 118°C and not over 12 pounds steam pressure. Alternately, carbohydrates are available in the form of differentiation disks that can be aseptically added to the plain tubed medium as needed. If differentiation disks are used, the base medium can be tubed and autoclaved at 121°C and 15 pounds steam pressure. Sterile, tubed CTA-sugars should be inoculated with a heavy inoculum, stabbing to a depth of approximately 2 mm below the medium surface. Fermentation is indicated by a color change in the medium from red to yellow.

Cycloserine Cefoxitin Fructose Agar (CCFA)

Cycloserine cefoxitin fructose agar is a selective differential medium useful in the isolation and identification of *Clostridium difficile* from stool specimens of patients suspected to have antibiotic-associated diarrhea with pseudomembranous colitis. The selective ingredients, cycloserine and cefoxitin antibiotics, inhibit the growth of intestinal normal flora by interfering with cell wall synthesis of both gram-positive and gram-negative bacteria. Although indigenous bacteria are inhibited, *C. difficile* is not. Although cycloserine and cefoxitin are incorporated for their selective properties, fructose and a pH indicator are included to confirm that the isolates can ferment this sugar.

Formulation and Preparation

Step 1: Base Medium.

Proteose peptone no. 2	40.0 g
Sodium orthophosphate	5.0 g
Potassium dihydrophosphate	1.0 g
Sodium chloride	2.0 g
Magnesium sulfate	0.1 g
Fructose	6.0 g
Neutral red (1% solution in ethanol)	3.0 mL
Sodium taurocholate	1.0 g
Agar	20.0 g
Distilled/deionized water	1 L

Mix ingredients and heat to dissolve. Dispense into 100-mL quantities and sterilize by autoclaving (121°C for 15 minutes).

Step 2: Complete Medium. Cool basal medium to 50°C, and add cycloserine base to a final concentration of 500 mg/mL and cefoxitin base to a final concentration of 16 mg/mL. Pour into Petri dishes. *Note:* A variation of this medium is made with mannitol rather than fructose and uses bromthymol blue indicator. A second variation adds egg yolk suspension, so lecithinase and lipase activities can be detected.

Decarboxylase Test Medium (Moeller)

Decarboxylase test medium with an incorporated amino acid is a differential medium useful in the identification of fermentative and nonfermentative gram-negative bacteria. The differential ingredient is one of three amino acids, lysine, arginine, or ornithine. Decarboxylation of the amino acid yields alkaline end products detected by a change in the color of an incorporated pH-sensitive dye.

Formulation and Preparation

Step 1: Basal Medium.

Pancreatic hydrolysate of gelatin (peptone)	5.0 g
Beef extract	5.0 g
Dextrose	0.5 g
Pyridoxal	5 mg
Cresol red	5 mg
Bromcresol purple	10 mg
Distilled/deionized water	1 L

Final pH 6.0 ± 0.2

Rehydrate commercially available dehydrated medium. If 1 L of basal medium is to be used to make all three test media, divide the basal medium into four 250-mL portions. Immediately dispense one portion into screw-cap tubes and sterilize by autoclaving (121°C for 15 minutes). The tubed basal medium (no amino acid) serves as a control for reading the reactions.

Step 2: Differential Medium. To the basal medium, add sufficient quantity of the desired L-amino acid to produce a final 1% concentration (10 g/L; 2.5 g/250 mL) or the DL-amino acid to produce a final 2% concentration. Addition of lysine or arginine does not affect the final pH; however, ornithine is a highly acidic amino acid, and its addition requires readjustment of the pH with 1 N NaOH before sterilization. Dispense differential medium into screw-cap tubes, and sterilize by autoclaving (121°C for 15 minutes). Sterile decarboxylase tubes and a control tube should be inoculated from a 24-hour slant culture using a loop. Inoculated tubes should be overlaid with 4 to 5 mm of sterile mineral oil to avoid oxidative deamination of available protein, which would falsely be interpreted as a positive reaction. Inoculated, overlaid tubes should be incubated at 35°C for up to 4 days. Incubating tubes should be checked daily. Fermentative organisms, early in the incubation, ferment glucose, turning the control and all decarboxylase tubes yellow. For these organisms, as the pH drops, the hydrogen ion concentration becomes optimal for decarboxylase activity. In the decarboxylase tubes, the subsequent conversion of the amino acid to amines raises the pH, reversing the yellow color to purple while the control tube remains yellow. Nonfermenters do not produce the initial yellow color change, and use of the amino acid is indicated by the amino acid–containing tube becoming a deeper purple than the control.

Deoxycholate Citrate Agar

Deoxycholate citrate agar is a selective differential medium useful in the isolation of enteric pathogens directly from feces and urine or indirectly from enrichment broths, such as Selenite-F. The selective ingredients are sodium citrate and sodium deoxycholate at concentrations that inhibit the majority of nonpathogenic enteric bacilli. The differential ingredient is lactose. Nonfermenter, enteric pathogens appear as colorless colonies. Those lactose-fermenters that do overcome the inhibitors appear as pink to red colonies as a result of the pH change accompanying lactose fermentation.

Formulation and Preparation

Infusion from 375 g of meat	10.0 g
Peptic digest of animal tissues (thiotone/proteose peptone)	10.0 g
Lactose	10.0 g
Sodium citrate	20.0 g
Sodium deoxycholate	5.0 g
Ferric citrate	1.0 g
Agar	17.0 g
Neutral red	20.0 mg
Distilled/deionized water	1 L

Final pH 7.3 ± 0.2

Rehydrate commercially available dehydrated medium according to manufacturer's directions, and heat, with frequent agitation, to boiling. Boil for 1 minute, cool to 45 to 50°C, and dispense into sterile Petri dishes. *Do not autoclave.* Allow plated medium to solidify with the lids ajar to prevent the condensation of excessive surface moisture. If plated medium appears wet, invert the plates and tilt the bottoms (containing agar) on the edges of the lids (inverted, ajar). Plates may be stored refrigerated for several days. Plated medium should be inoculated, streaked for isolation, and incubated at 35°C in air (not in CO_2) for up to 48 hours. A heavy inoculum is recommended if the specimen is feces, urine, or other direct bodily materials, whereas a light inoculum is recommended if one is subculturing from an initial enrichment broth.

Deoxyribonuclease (DNase) Test Agar (With/Without Indicator Dye)

DNase test agar is a differential medium used to detect the production of an active DNase exoenzyme by aerobic bacterial species. The differential ingredient is incorporated DNA. Methods available for detection of DNA degradation include hydrochloric acid precipitation of undegraded DNA and color change of an incorporated metachromatic dye such as toluidine blue or methyl green.

Formulation and Preparation

Step 1: Base Medium.

Papaic digest of soybean meal	5.0 g
Pancreatic digest of casein	15.0 g
DNA	2.0 g
Sodium chloride	5.0 g
Agar	15.0 g
Distilled/deionized water	1 L

Step 2: Optional Ingredients (to be used if metachromatic dyes are to be used in detection of DNA degradation).

Metachromatic dye: toluidine blue   100 mg
                    or
Metachromatic dye: methyl green   50 mg

Step 3: Developer Reagent (1 N HCl to be used if HCl precipitation is used to detect DNA degradation).

HCl, concentrated   2.8 mL
Distilled/deionized water   97.2 mL

Rehydrate commercially available dehydrated agar, either basal or with incorporated metachromatic dye, according to manufacturer's directions. Sterilize by autoclaving (121°C for 15 minutes), and dispense into sterile Petri dishes. Sterile, plated medium should be inoculated using a 1 to 2-cm streak or an approximately 5-mm diameter spot inoculum. Inoculated plates should be incubated aerobically at 35°C for 18 to 24 hours. Following incubation, DNase activity is detected in one of the following ways:

1. If basal medium without a metachromatic dye was inoculated, flood the plate with 1 N HCl and look for a zone of clearing around the bacterial growth. If the incorporated DNA is undegraded, it is precipitated by the 1 N HCl and the medium becomes opaque. If the incorporated DNA is degraded, the nucleotide fragments dissolve in the 1 N HCl and the medium remains clear.

2. If the medium included toluidine blue, the blue DNA-bound dye is released from nucleotide fragments, producing a color change to rose. The medium remains clear blue in negative reactions.

3. If the medium included methyl green, the green DNA-bound dye is released from nucleotide fragments, resulting in a loss of color. The medium remains green in negative reactions.

E Medium, Diphasic

E medium is one of many media developed for the isolation and culture of mycoplasmal organisms. This medium is enriched with a yeast dialysate, horse serum, penicillin, and thallium acetate.

Formulation and Preparation

Step 1: Yeast Dialysate. Suspend 450 g of active dried yeast, such as Fleischman's, in 1,250 mL of distilled/deionized water at 40°C and autoclave at 121°C for 5 minutes. Place in a dialysis casing, and dialyze refrigerated against 1 L of distilled/deionized water for 48 hours. Autoclave dialysate (121°C for 15 minutes) and store frozen.

Step 2: E Agar.

Papaic digest of soy meal   20.0 g
Sodium chloride   5.0 g

Purified water	1.0 L
Agar	10.0 g

Mix ingredients, and heat while agitating gently to put ingredients into solution. Cool the solution, and adjust the pH to 7.4 with 1 N sodium hydroxide. Aliquot basal agar in 65-mL portions, and sterilize by autoclaving (121°C for 15 minutes). Any basal medium not used immediately can be stored refrigerated and remelted for use as needed. Cool media aliquots to 50°C. To each 65-mL aliquot add 10 mL of yeast dialysate, 25 mL of sterile horse serum, 2 mL of penicillin (20,000 units), and 1 mL of 3.3% aqueous thallium acetate. Completed agar may be dispensed in 3-mL quantities into 16×125 mm screw-capped tubes or in 5-mL amounts into 10×35 mm Petri dishes and allowed to solidify.

Step 3: E Broth.

Papaic digest of soy meal	20.0 g
Sodium chloride	5.0 g
Dextrose	10.0 g
Purified water	1.0 L
Phenol red, 2% aqueous	2.0 mL

Dissolve all ingredients, and adjust to pH 7.6. Dispense into 65-mL aliquots, and sterilize by autoclaving (121°C for 15 minutes). Cool, and to each aliquot add 10 mL of yeast dialysate, 25 mL of sterile horse serum, 2 mL of penicillin (20,000 units), and 1 mL of 3.3% aqueous thallium acetate.

Step 4: Diphasic E Medium. Overlay tubed E agar with 3 mL of E broth, and store at room temperature. *Caution:* Tubes must be tightly capped to prevent loss of CO_2 from incorporated horse serum, resulting in elevation of the medium pH.

Egg Yolk Agar, CDC Formulation (EYA)

Egg yolk agar is a differential medium useful in the detection of lecithinase, lipase, and protease activity. Incorporated egg emulsion provides the lecithin, lipids, and proteins to be degraded by these enzymes. On egg yolk agar, exoenzyme activity is detected as follows: Lecithinase activity produces a zone of opacity immediately around the growth streak; lipase activity results in an iridescent sheen on or around the surface of colonies; protease activity is seen as a clearing of the medium around and just beyond the streaked growth area. A given organism may produce one or all of these exoenzymes.

Formulation and Preparation

Step 1: Basal Medium.

Pancreatic digest of casein	40.0 g
NaHPO$_4$	5.0 g
MgSO$_4$ (5% aqueous solution)	0.2 mL
Yeast extract	5.0 g
D-glucose	2.0 g
Sodium chloride	2.0 g

Agar	25.0 g
Distilled/deionized water	900 mL

Mix and dissolve all ingredients by heating to boiling, and sterilize by autoclaving (121°C for 15 minutes).

Step 2: Complete Medium (Final pH 7.4). Cool basal medium to 50°C, and add 100 mL of commercial or laboratory-made egg yolk emulsion, mix, dispense into Petri plates, and allow to cool with lids ajar to minimize surface moisture. Plated medium should be inoculated as single streak across the plate and incubated anaerobically at 35°C for 24 to 72 hours. *Note:* If the Nagler test is to be performed, one half of the plate surface should be smeared with a few drops of *C. perfringens* type A antitoxin before inoculation. The inoculation streak should then extend across both halves (no antitoxin/antitoxin) of the plate. Inoculated plates should be incubated anaerobically at 35°C for 24 to 48 hours. A positive test result is the inhibition of lecithinase activity on the half of the plate with antitoxin. Plated medium not used immediately may be stored at 4°C if sealed in plastic bags.

Eosin-Methylene Blue Agar (EMB)

Eosin-methylene blue agar is a selective differential medium useful in the isolation and identification of gram-negative enteric bacteria. Eosin Y and methylene blue dyes, the selective ingredients, are incorporated to inhibit the growth of gram-positive bacteria while allowing the growth of gram-negative bacteria. The carbohydrates lactose and sucrose are incorporated to allow differentiation of isolates based on lactose fermentation. Fermentation is detected by color changes and precipitation of the incorporated dyes as the pH drops. Sucrose serves as an alternative carbohydrate source for slow lactose fermenters, allowing their timely elimination from consideration as possible pathogens. *Escherichia coli,* a coliform lactose fermenter, typically forms blue-black colonies with a metallic greenish sheen. Other coliform fermenters, such as *Enterobacter,* form pink colonies. Nonfermenter colonies are translucent, being either amber colored or colorless.

Formulation and Preparation

Pancreatic hydrolysate of gelatin	10.0 g
Lactose	5.0 g
Sucrose	5.0 g
Dipotassium phosphate	2.0 g
Eosin Y	0.4 g
Methylene blue	65 mg
Agar	13.5 g
Distilled/deionized water	1 L

Rehydrate commercially available dehydrated medium according to manufacturer's directions, and sterilize by autoclaving (121°C for 15 minutes). Following autoclaving, the methylene blue dye is reduced and appears orange. The flask of autoclaved medium should be gently agitated to restore the methylene blue to its oxidized form (purple color) and poured into sterile Petri dishes. Plated medium should be allowed to cool with lids ajar to avoid the collection of excessive surface moisture. Cooled, plated medium should be inoculated, streaked for isolation, and incubated aerobically (not in CO_2) at 35°C for 18 to 24 hours.

Esculin Agar

Esculin agar is a differential medium used to determine the ability of an organism to hydrolyze esculin. The hydrolytic products from esculin react with the ferric salt present in this medium to precipitate iron compounds and produce a gray-to-black discoloration of the medium.

Formulation and Preparation

Esculin	1.0 g
Ferric citrate	0.5 g
Heart infusion agar	40.0 g
Distilled/deionized water	1 L

Mix ingredients, and heat to dissolve. Cool to 55°C, and adjust to pH 7.0. Dispense as 5-mL quantities into 16 × 125 mm tubes, cotton-plug, and sterilize by autoclaving (121°C for 15 minutes). Cool in a slanted position. Slanted medium should be inoculated, incubated aerobically at 35°C, and observed for growth, with darkening of the medium indicative of esculin hydrolysis.

Fletcher Semisolid Medium for Leptospira

Fletcher semisolid medium is an enrichment medium recommended for detection of leptospiral species in blood, spinal fluid, and urine specimens as well as possibly contaminated water and other materials. The enrichment component of this medium is rabbit serum containing some hemoglobin.

Formulation and Preparation

Step 1: Base Medium.

Pancreatic hydrolysate of gelatin, *USP*	0.3 g
Beef extract	0.2 g
Sodium chloride	0.5 g
Agar	1.5 g
Distilled/deionized water	920 mL
Final pH 7.9 ± 1	

Rehydrate commercially available base medium according to manufacturer's directions. Mix and heat to boiling to dissolve completely; sterilize by autoclaving (121°C for 15 minutes).

Step 2: Complete Medium. Cool sterile base medium to 50 to 55°C, and add 80 mL of rabbit serum with natural hemoglobin. Lyophilized rabbit serum with natural hemoglobin is commercially available as Leptospira Enrichment (Difco, Detroit MI), or sterile, pooled fresh natural rabbit serum may be added. Aseptically dispense into sterile screw-cap tubes, 5 mL/tube, and store at room temperature overnight. The complete medium must be inactivated by placing tubes in a 56°C water bath for 1 hour on the day following preparation. Cooled inactivated medium should be inoculated with a drop or two of the fluid specimen using a sterile, plugged Pasteur pipette. Small inocula introduced into multiple tubes are recommended to optimize pathogen recovery and minimize any interference by developing antibody titers in the body fluid specimens. Inoculated tubes should be incubated with caps loose at 25 to 30°C for 4 to 5 weeks and examined weekly for growth in the form of turbidity at the top of the medium. A loopful of fluid from any tube showing turbidity should be placed on a clean slide, coverslipped, and examined by darkfield microscopy.

Gelatin Medium (Nutrient)

Gelatin medium is a differential medium used to determine a bacterial isolate's ability to produce gelatinase and thereby hydrolyze gelatin. A variety of gelatin-containing media can be used for this purpose, including starch-gelatin agar, Kohn modified gelation for the Kohn gelatin method, and nutrient gelatin.

Formulation and Preparation

Pancreatic hydrolysate of gelatin, *USP*	5.0 g
Beef extract	3.0 g
Gelatin	120.0 g
Distilled/deionized water	1 L
Final pH 6.8	

Rehydrate commercially available dehydrated medium according to manufacturer's directions, dispense into tubes, and sterilize by autoclaving (121°C for 15 minutes). Sterile, tubed medium can be stored at 4°C. Sterile tubed medium is inoculated and incubated, with an uninoculated control tube, at 35°C for 18 to 24 hours. Following incubation, both the inoculated and the control tube are refrigerated for 30 minutes before reading. The control tube should gel, whereas the inoculated tube consistency depends on the isolate's ability or inability to hydrolyze gelatin. If the inoculated tube gels, the isolate in question is gelatinase negative. If the gelatin in the inoculated tube remains liquid, the isolate in question is gelatinase positive.

Gram-Negative Broth

Gram-negative broth is an enrichment-selective medium used to enhance the chance of recovering enteric pathogens, such as *Salmonella* and *Shigella* species, from fecal specimens. The selective ingredients are deoxycholate and citrate salts that retard the growth of gram-positive bacteria, while allowing the growth of aerobic gram-negative bacteria. Enrichment is provided by increasing the concentration of mannitol, which favors, temporarily, the growth of mannitol-fermenting, gram-negative rods over that of the mannitol nonfermenters.

Formulation and Preparation

Pancreatic digest of casein, *USP*	10.0 g
Peptic digest of animal tissue, *USP*	10.0 g
D-Glucose	1.0 g
D-Mannitol	2.0 g
Sodium citrate	5.0 g
Sodium deoxycholate	0.5 g
Dipotassium phosphate	4.0 g
Monopotassium phosphate	1.5 g
Sodium chloride	5.0 g
Distilled/deionized water	1 L

Final pH 7.0 ± 0.2

Rehydrate commercially available dehydrated medium according to manufacturer's directions, heat to boiling, dispense into test tubes, and sterilize capped tubes by autoclaving (116°C for 15 minutes). Sterile, tubed medium should be inoculated with fecal material and incubated, with caps loosened, at 35°C. Incubated gram-negative broth cultures should be subcultured onto selective differential plated media after 6 to 8 hours and again after 18 to 24 hours.

Hektoen Enteric Agar (HE)

Hektoen enteric agar is a selective differential medium used for direct isolation of enteric pathogens from feces and for indirect isolation from selective-enrichment broth. The selective ingredients are bile salts at concentrations that not only inhibit the growth of gram-positive bacteria, but also retard the growth of many normal intestinal flora gram-negative organisms. The differential ingredients include lactose and sucrose, to determine fermentation patterns, and ferric salts, to detect the production of hydrogen sulfide gas.

Formulation and Preparation

Peptic digest of animal tissue, *USP*	12.0 g
Yeast extract	3.0 g
Bile salts	9.0 g
Lactose	12.0 g
Sucrose	12.0 g
Salicin	2.0 g
Sodium thiosulfate	5.0 g

Ferric ammonium citrate	1.5 g
Sodium chloride	5.0 g
Acid-fuchsin	190 mg
Bromthymol blue	65 mg
Agar	14.0 g
Distilled/deionized water	1 L

Final pH 7.5 ± 0.2

Rehydrate commercially available dehydrated medium according to manufacturer's directions, and heat just to boiling to dissolve completely. *Avoid overheating, and do not autoclave.* Dispense into sterile Petri dishes, and allow the medium to set up with lids ajar to prevent excessive surface moisture. Plated medium should be inoculated, streaked for isolation, and incubated aerobically (not in CO_2) at 35°C for 18 to 24 hours. Most nonpathogens ferment one or both of the sugars, and colonies appear bright orange to salmon-pink in color owing to the low pH interaction with incorporated dyes. Nonfermenters, such as *Salmonella* and *Shigella* species, typically produce green to blue-green appearing colonies. Hydrogen sulfide gas production is seen as a black precipitate that accumulates within colonies.

Hippurate Broth

Hippurate broth is a differential broth useful in the identification of group B streptococci. The differential ingredient is 1% sodium hippurate, which the group B streptococci hydrolyze to glycine and benzoic acid. Hydrolysis, in this method, is detected by the addition of ferric chloride, which reacts with the benzoic acid to produce ferric benzoate, which precipitates.

Formulation and Preparation

| Heart infusion broth | 1 L |
| Sodium hippurate | 1.0 g |

Rehydrate commercially available heart infusion broth according to manufacturer's directions, add and dissolve the sodium hippurate, dispense as 2-mL quantities into tubes, and sterilize by autoclaving (121°C for 15 minutes). Sterile, tubed medium should be inoculated and incubated, along with an uninoculated control tube, at 35°C for 48 hours. Following incubation, 12% ferric chloride is added a drop at a time to the control tube. A precipitate forms initially but dissolves as one continues to add ferric chloride. Count the total number of drops added to the control tube by the time the precipitate redissolves. Add that number of drops to the inoculated tube. A positive reaction is grossly visible precipitate that persists 10 minutes or longer after the addition of ferric chloride. A negative reaction yields no precipitate or a faint precipitate, which disappears in less than 10 minutes after the addition of ferric chloride.

Note: A rapid method available uses a 1% aqueous solution of sodium hippurate dispensed in 0.4-mL quantities. Colonies of the isolate are emulsified in the solution until it is cloudy and incubated in a 37°C water bath for 2 hours. Hydrolysis is detected by adding five drops of triketohydrindene hydrate

(Ninhydrin) reagent (without shaking the tube) and continuing to incubate for a minimum of 10 but not longer than 30 minutes. Positive reactions are deep purple in color, whereas negative reactions show no color change.

Hydrogen Sulfide, Lead Acetate

Lead acetate is one differential method used to detect the production of H_2S from sulfur-containing amino acids. The organism is cultured in a nutrient broth or on an agar medium with sufficient protein to ensure the presence of sulfur-containing amino acids. As the organism metabolizes these amino acids, H_2S gas is evolved. The liberated gas is detected by lead acetate–impregnated paper strips that are suspended over the culture during incubation. The produced H_2S reacts with the lead acetate to produce lead sulfide, a black insoluble salt, causing the strip to blacken. Lead acetate strips are available commercially.

Kligler Iron Agar

Purpose

Kligler iron agar (KIA) can be used to determine if a gram-negative rod is a glucose fermenter or nonfermenter, a fundamental characteristic in the initial classification of gram-negative rods. The medium also tests for lactose fermentation, gas production during carbohydrate fermentation, and hydrogen sulfide production, all of which are useful in the differentiation of gram-negative rods belonging to the family *Enterobacteriaceae*.

Principle

KIA contains glucose and lactose (fermentable carbohydrates), phenol red (pH indicator), peptone (carbon/nitrogen source), and iron salt plus sodium thiosulfate (sulfur source and hydrogen sulfide indicator). KIA resembles triple sugar iron agar except it lacks sucrose. Three carbohydrate fermentation patterns are possible:

1. Acid (yellow) butt and alkaline (red) slant indicate that the organism ferments glucose but not lactose. This organism ferments glucose by Embden-Meyerhof pathway to produce organic acids, changing the pH indicator from red to yellow. Once the glucose has been consumed, the organism then breaks down peptones, producing ammonia. This causes a pH rise and reverts the slant to red.

2. Acid (yellow) butt and acid (yellow) slant indicate that the organism ferments both glucose and lactose. The organism ferments glucose, producing acid products. Once the glucose is consumed, it ferments lactose, breaking it down into glucose and galactose. This causes the pH in the slant portion to remain acidic.

3. Alkaline (red) butt and alkaline (red) slant indicate that the organism cannot ferment glucose or lactose and therefore produces no acidic products. The slant may become more red because of peptone catabolism.

If there are gas bubbles in butt, splitting of the medium, or displacement of medium from bottom of tube, the organism is aerogenic—able to produce carbon dioxide and hydrogen gases during fermentation. Any blackening in the butt indicates that the organism produces hydrogen sulfide gas from thiosulfate. The hydrogen sulfide combines with iron salt to produce ferrous sulfide, a black precipitate.

Formulation

Two formulations (BBL and Difco), available as powdered media, are in common use. Note that the Difco formulation includes yeast and meat extracts and uses ferrous sulfate rather than ferric ammonium citrate.

Peptone or polypeptone	20.000 g
Meat extract (optional)	3.000 g
Yeast extract (optional)	3.000 g
Lactose	10.000 g
Glucose	1.000 g
Sodium chloride	5.000 g
Ferric ammonium citrate	0.500 g
Sodium thiosulfate	0.500 g
Agar	12 to 15.000 g
Phenol red	0.025 g
Distilled water	1.000 L
Final pH 7.4	

Preparation and Special Considerations

Ingredients should be mixed with heat and agitation, dispensed into tubes, and autoclaved at 121°C for 15 minutes at 15 lb pressure. Tubes should be cooled in slanted position. For optimal detection of reactions, it is important that butt be deep and approximately the same length as slant. Final medium should be red. Inoculation is done by stabbing the butt with the inoculating needle and streaking the slant using pure culture of isolate. The cap should be slightly loose. If the cap is screwed on too tightly, there will not be sufficient air for peptone catabolism. Gram-negative rods able to ferment glucose only may appear as lactose fermenters. Reactions should be interpreted at 18 to 24 hours. If read earlier, organisms able to ferment glucose only may appear to be lactose fermenters. If read later, lactose fermenters may consume the lactose and begin to catabolize peptones, reverting slant to red color. A yellow slant and red butt may indicate failure to stab butt or inoculation of medium with gram-positive organism. Examination of medium for stab line or performance of Gram stain should clarify this situation. Hydrogen sulfide indicator system in KIA is not as sensitive as the lead acetate method or as that found in other media, such as sulfide indole motility agar. A black butt should be read as acid even though yellow color may be obscured. If hydrogen sulfide is reduced, this indicates that an acid condition does exist and can be assumed. Critical to understanding how this medium works is the fact that glucose is present in much lesser amount than lactose. Organisms use the simplest carbohydrate, glucose, first. Once this is consumed, they attack the more complex carbohydrate, lactose. If they lack the appropriate enzymes, they move on to protein catabolism. There is sufficient lactose in the medium to prevent breakdown of peptone, provided that it is read at the appropriate time.

Loeffler Coagulated Serum Slant

Purpose

Loeffler coagulated serum slant is primarily used for recovery and identification of *Corynebacterium diphtheriae*. Other uses include detection of proteolysis, pigment formation, and ascospore production as well as cultivation of *Entamoeba histolytica*.

Principle

This medium can be used for primary recovery of *C. diphtheriae* from nose and throat specimens and for subculture purposes. Because Loeffler medium is so enriched, *C. diphtheriae* grows well within 12 to 16 hours and produces nondistinctive translucent to gray-white colonies. The medium promotes the development of characteristic granules that can be detected microscopically with methylene blue stains. Serum content enables detection of proteolytic activity. Positive organisms produce colonies surrounded by small holes containing liquefied medium. The entire slant may eventually turn to liquid with production of a foul odor.

Formulation

Several formulations are available. The one listed is an adaptation from BBL. The Difco formulation consists of three parts volume of beef, hog, or horse blood serum and one part volume of glucose infusion broth with no egg.

Beef serum (dry solids)	70.0 g
Sodium chloride	0.4 g
D-Glucose	0.7 g
Peptic digest of casein	0.7 g
Pancreatic digest of heart muscle	0.7 g
Egg (whole, dried)	7.5 g
Distilled water	1.0 L
Final pH 7.6	

Preparation and Special Considerations

Loeffler coagulated serum slants are difficult to make, and most microbiologists prefer purchasing the medium in prepared form. The medium is rehydrated, heated to 45°C, and gently mixed to avoid production of air bubbles. The suspension is dispensed into tubes. Because of heat-sensitive components such as egg, the tubed medium is sterilized in the autoclave by inspissation. Tubes are placed in slanted position and exposed to 70°C for 6 hours on 3 successive days. To prevent the formation of a bumpy surface, temperature should be elevated slowly. This keeps the serum on the surface from coagulating before air is driven out of the medium. The final medium should be smooth and grayish white and in slants.

Loeffler serum slant should be inoculated as soon as possible after specimen collection, and more selective media containing tellurite should always be used as well. Smears for *C. diphtheriae* should be prepared and examined after 8 to 24 hours of incubation. Although granule formation is typical of *Corynebacterium* species, other organisms can produce a similar microscopic appearance. Therefore, additional testing must be performed for confirmation of this organism. Proteolysis testing may require 3 to 4 days of aerobic incubation or longer. For ascospore detection, the slants must be dried out. Excess liquid should be poured out of the tube. Slant may be heated until it splits. Screwed caps can be replaced with cotton plug to maintain a drier environment. Ascospores tend to form on drier areas of the medium.

Löwenstein-Jensen Medium (LJ)

Purpose

Löwenstein-Jensen medium is used to cultivate *Mycobacterium* species.

Principle

Most media contain ingredients that can inhibit the growth of mycobacteria. The potato flour, egg, and glycerol included in LJ medium help detoxify this medium and also supply nutrients required for growth of these organisms. Asparagine is included for maximum production of niacin by certain *Mycobacterium* species. The malachite green serves as an inhibitor of other bacteria that may be present in specimens.

Formulation

Basal Medium.

Monopotassium phosphate, anhydrous	2.40 g
Magnesium sulfate	0.24 g
Magnesium citrate	0.60 g
Asparagine	3.60 g
Potato flour	30.00 g
Glycerol, reagent grade	12.00 mL
Distilled water	600.00 mL

Additives.

Homogenized whole eggs	1000.00 mL
Malachite green, 2% aqueous	20.00 mL

Preparation and Special Considerations

Basal medium is prepared by dissolving salts and asparagine in water followed by addition of glycerol and potato flour. Basal medium is autoclaved at 121°C for 30 minutes and cooled to room temperature. Homogenized egg suspension is prepared by scrubbing eggs (1 week or less in age) with 5% soap solution. The eggs are thoroughly rinsed in cold running water and then placed for 15 minutes in 70% ethanol. The treated eggs are broken into a sterile flask and homogenized by hand shaking the flask. Sterile glass beads may be added to enhance the process. The resulting suspension is filtered through four layers of sterile gauze. After addition of homogenized eggs and malachite green solution to basal medium, the medium is dispensed into tubes and inspissated in slanted position at 85°C for 50 minutes. It is important to check the medium for sterility by incubating at 35 to 37°C for 48 hours. LJ medium is good for one month if tightly capped to prevent moisture loss and stored at 4 to 6°C. LJ medium must be kept out of direct light because malachite green is light sensitive. Decontaminated/digested or untreated specimens are inoculated onto medium and incubated in carbon dioxide incubator (5 to 10% CO_2) for 6 to 10 weeks. It is important to leave caps loose for proper gas exchange.

LJ medium may be prepared as deeps to be used in the semiquantitative catalase test for speciation of *Mycobacterium* species. LJ medium with 5% sodium chloride may be prepared to aid in the speciation of rapid growers. This medium is the same as LJ except for addition of 5 g sodium chloride per each 100 mL medium. The additional salt allows for testing the ability of certain mycobacteria to tolerate and grow in the presence of high salt concentration. The Gruft modification makes this medium more selective through the addition of penicillin (50 units/mL) and nalidixic acid (35 μg/mL) before dispensing into tubes. This formulation also includes 0.05 μg/mL ribonucleic acid, which increases the rate of mycobacterium isolation over standard LJ formulation. In the Petran and Vera modification, cyclohexamide, lincomycin, and nalidixic acid are added to make LJ more selective. Both of these modifications can permit gentler decontamination/digestion procedures.

Lysine-Iron Agar

Purpose

This medium measures three parameters useful in speciation of *Enterobacteriaceae:* lysine decarboxylation, lysine deamination, and hydrogen sulfide production.

Principle

Lysine-iron agar (LIA) contains lysine (amino acid), glucose (carbohydrate source), a small amount of protein, bromcresol purple (pH indicator), and sodium thiosulfate/ferric ammonium citrate (sulfur source and hydrogen sulfide indicator).

Three lysine utilization patterns are possible:

1. Alkaline (purple) butt and alkaline (purple) slant indicate that the organism decarboxylates lysine but cannot deaminate it. Initially the organism ferments glucose, causing production of acid and changing indicator in butt to yellow. It then decarboxylates lysine to produce cadaverine, an alkaline product. This causes the pH indicator to change back to purple.

2. Acid (yellow) butt and alkaline (purple) slant indicate that the organism fermented the glucose but was unable to deaminate or decarboxylate the lysine.

3. Acid (yellow) butt and Bordeaux red slant indicate that the organism deaminated lysine but could not decarboxylate it. The yellow butt is caused by glucose fermentation. The reason for red slant in cases of lysine deamination has not been clarified. If no indicator is present, one of the products of deamination appears orange. The red slant may be the result of mixing purple and red colors.

Any blackening in butt indicates production of hydrogen sulfide from sodium thiosulfate. This gas reacts with ferric salt to produce the black precipitate, ferrous sulfide.

Formulation

Peptone	5.0 g
Yeast extract	3.0 g
D-Glucose	1.0 g
L-Lysine hydrochloride	10.0 g
Ferric ammonium citrate	0.5 g
Sodium thiosulfate	40.0 mg
Bromcresol purple	20.0 mg
Agar	13.5 to 15.0 g
Distilled water	1.0 L
Final pH 6.7	

Preparation and Special Considerations

Ingredients are mixed in water and heated to boiling. The medium is dispensed into tubes and autoclaved at 121°C for 12 to 15 minutes. Tubes are cooled in a slanted position to form short slants and deep butts. This medium appears purple before use. LIA is inoculated by stabbing butt twice and streaking slant with an inoculating needle. Cap should be left slightly loose because oxygen is required for detection of deamination. Reactions should be read after 18 to 24 hours of incubation at 35°C. The medium may be incubated up to 48 hours if needed.

LIA is not as sensitive as other media for hydrogen sulfide detection. Typically, hydrogen sulfide–producing *Proteus* species may appear negative. Also, *Morganella morganii* produces variable lysine deamination reaction after 24 hours' incubation. This medium can only be used with organisms that can ferment glucose. LIA is not a true replacement for the Moeller decarboxylase tests.

MacConkey Agar

Purpose

MacConkey agar is a selective differential primary plating medium. It selects for *Enterobacteriaceae* and other gram-negative rods in the presence of mixed flora and differentiates them into lactose fermenters and nonfermenters.

Principle

Bile salts and crystal violet inhibit most gram-positive organisms but permit the growth of gram-negative rods. Lactose serves as the sole carbohydrate source. Gram-negative rods that ferment lactose produce pink or red colonies, which may be surrounded by precipitated bile. Acid production from lactose fermentation causes the neutral dye absorbed into the colonies to change to red and can also cause the bile salts to become insoluble. Non–lactose-fermenting, gram-negative rods produce colorless or transparent colonies.

Formulation

Peptone (pancreatic hydrolysate of gelatin)	17.0 g
Polypeptone (pancreatic hydrolysate of casein and peptic digest of animal tissue)	3.0 g
Lactose	10.0 g
Bile salts	1.5 g
Sodium chloride	5.0 g
Agar	13.5 to 15.0 g
Neutral red	30.0 mg
Crystal violet	1.0 mg
Distilled water	1.0 L
Final pH 7.1	

Preparation and Special Considerations

Ingredients should be mixed in water and heated to boiling. The medium is then autoclaved at 121°C for 15 minutes, cooled to 45°C, and poured into Petri dishes. Lids should be left ajar during cooling to prevent excess moisture accumulation on the surface. Plates are streaked for isolation and incubated in ambient air, not carbon dioxide incubator, for 18 to 24 hours at 35°C. Weak or slow lactose fermenters may produce colorless colonies at 24 hours or appear slightly pink in 24 to 48 hours. Plates should not be incubated longer than 48 hours because this can lead to confusing results. Some gram-negative rods may fail to grow on the medium, whereas with prolonged incubation, gram-positive cocci such as *Enterococcus* species may produce tiny colonies. Room temperature incubation may enhance recovery of *Yersinia enterocolitica.*

Agar concentration may be increased to prevent swarming of *Proteus* species. A formulation of MacConkey agar without crystal violet has been used to aid in speciation of mycobacteria. A closely related medium, MacConkey sorbitol agar, contains the same components as regular MacConkey agar except D-sorbitol is substituted for lactose. This medium has been used for isolating *E. coli* 0157:H7. Sorbitol-negative colonies, which appear colorless on this medium, may indicate possible *E. coli* 0157:H7 and should be further tested.

Malonate Broth

Purpose

Malonate broth is used in the identification of *Enterobacteriaceae,* particularly in the speciation of *Salmonella.*

Principle

Malonate broth contains sodium malonate (primary carbon source), small quantities of glucose and yeast extract (nutrients), bromthymol blue (pH indicator), various salts, and a buffering system. Organisms producing a Prussian blue color are able to use malonate as a carbon source. If they can use malonate as a carbon source, they also employ ammonium sulfate as a nitrogen source, thereby producing alkaline products that cause a pH rise and change in medium color to blue. Organisms unable to use malonate as a carbon source usually fail to grow, and the medium stays green. Because malonate resembles succinate, it competitively binds succinic dehydrogenase, which catalyzes the succinate to fumarate conversion in the Krebs cycle. The tying up of this enzyme, coupled with inability to use malonate as a carbon source, prevents growth.

Formulation

Yeast extract	1.000 g
Ammonium sulfate	2.000 g
Dipotassium sulfate	0.600 g
Monopotassium sulfate	0.400 g
Sodium chloride	2.000 g
Sodium malonate	3.000 g
Glucose	0.250 g
Bromthymol blue	0.025 g
Distilled water	1.000 L
Final pH 6.7	

Preparation and Special Considerations

The ingredients are mixed in water, heated to boiling, and distributed into tubes. The medium is then autoclaved at 121°C for 15 minutes. Malonate broth should be inoculated from triple sugar iron agar, KIA, or broth culture of the organism. Inoculum should be light. Cultures should be incubated at 35°C and checked at 18 to 24 hours and at 48 hours for production of blue color. Some organisms produce only small amounts of alkalinity. Any trace of blue should be considered positive. Comparison with an uninoculated tube may be useful. Production of a yellow color is a negative reaction. This is probably due to fermentation of the small amount of glucose in the medium.

Mannitol Salt Agar

Purpose

Mannitol salt agar is a selective differential primary culture medium useful in recovery and identification of staphylococci from specimens containing mixed flora.

Principle

High salt concentration (7.5%) inhibits most gram-negative rods and gram-positive rods except *Staphylococcus* species. *Staphylococcus aureus* is able to ferment mannitol, the sole carbohydrate in the medium, to produce acid products. This lowers the pH and changes the color of the pH indicator, phenol red, to yellow. Colonies of *S. aureus* typically appear yellow surrounded by a yellow zone. Other *Staphylococcus* species and *Micrococcus* species usually do not ferment mannitol and therefore produce reddish colonies, which may exhibit a red-to-purple surrounding zone owing to peptone breakdown.

Formulation

Beef extract	1.000 g
Peptone or polypeptone (pancreatic digest of casein and peptic digest of animal tissue)	10.000 g
Sodium chloride	75.000 g
Mannitol	10.000 g
Agar	15.000 g
Phenol red	0.025 g
Distilled water	1.000 L
Final pH 7.4	

Preparation and Special Considerations

Ingredients are dissolved in water by heating. Medium is autoclaved at 121°C for 15 minutes, cooled to 48°C, and poured into plates. Plates are streaked for isolation and incubated at 35°C for 24 to 48 hours but not in carbon dioxide incubator. *Enterococcus* may be able to grow on mannitol salt agar and produce slight mannitol fermentation. Differentiation is readily accomplished through Gram stain and catalase test. With prolonged incubation, organisms other than staphylococci may begin to grow and produce mannitol fermentation. Some strains of *S. aureus* may be slow in fermenting mannitol, so plates should not be discarded until after 48 hours of incubation. All colonies suggestive of *S. aureus* should be further tested by coagulase or an acceptable alternative procedure. Subculture to less selective agar is preferable before performing this testing. Some formulations recommend inclusion of 20 mL sterile egg yolk. Coagulase-positive staphylococci also produce a lipase that causes formation of opaque precipitate around the colonies. Non–coagulase-producing staphylococci do not produce this egg yolk lipase and therefore lack these zones.

MES (Ureaplasma Agar)

Purpose

MES agar is used for the isolation of *Ureaplasma urealyticum*.

Principle

This medium contains horse serum, which supplies the cholesterol necessary for stabilizing these organisms because they lack cell walls. Yeast dialysate serves as a growth factor and supplies preformed nucleic acid precursors. Urea is a required nutrient for *Ureaplasma*. Phenol red serves as a pH indicator, whereas MES or 2-(N-Morpholino) ethanesulfonic acid acts as a buffer. The antibiotics, penicillin and lincomycin, inhibit normal flora but permit the growth of *Ureaplasma*.

Formulation

Agar basal medium (heat and cool to 50°C before use; see next)	70	mL
Yeast dialysate (see next)	10	mL
Sterile horse serum	20	mL
1 M urea (see next)	0.2	mL
Penicillin stock solution (see next)	1	mL
Lincomycin solution (prepare fresh, 10,000 μg/mL)	0.5	mL

Preparation of solutions used in the formulation is as follows:

1. MES buffer

2-(N-Morpholino) ethanesulfonic acid	195 g
Water, distilled	800 mL

   Adjust pH to 6.0 with concentrated sodium hydroxide. Adjust final volume to 1,000 mL. Use a membrane filter to sterilize the solution. Buffer should be stored away from light at room temperature.

2. 1% phenol red

Phenol red   1 g
Water, distilled   100 mL
Solution should be autoclaved at 121°C for 15 minutes.

3. 1 molar urea

Urea   60 g
Water, distilled   100 mL
Dissolve urea in water and filter sterilize. Store at room temperature.

4. Penicillin stock solution

Penicillin G   1,000,000 U
Water, sterile   50 mL
Store in freezer.

5. Agar basal medium

Soy peptone   20   g
Sodium chloride   5   g
MES buffer   4.25 g
Phenol red (1%)   1   mL
Water, distilled   1,000 mL
Agar   10   g

6. Yeast dialysate

Bakers' yeast   908 g
Distilled water   1,000 mL
Make a smooth paste and autoclave at 121°C for 10 minutes. Cool; place in dialysis tubing, and dialyze against 2 L of cold distilled water. Collect dialysate; aliquot and store in freezer indefinitely.

Preparation and Special Considerations

After mixing components, pour medium into Petri dishes, 5 mL per plate. Store plates in plastic up to 2 weeks in refrigerator. Plates should be inoculated with 0.1 mL of specimen and incubated in a carbon dioxide incubator, in a candle jar, or under anaerobic conditions. At 48 hours, colonies of *Ureaplasma* show a "fried-egg" appearance. If a solution of 1% urea/0.8% manganese chloride is poured over these colonies, they turn dark brown owing to the production of urease.

Methyl Red–Voges-Proskauer Medium (MRVP)

Purpose

MRVP broth is used for performing the methyl red and Voges-Proskauer tests. These procedures are useful in distinguishing among members of the *Enterobacteriaceae*. For example, *E. coli* is methyl red positive and Voges-Proskauer negative; *Enterobacter aerogenes, Enterobacter cloacae,* and *Klebsiella pneumoniae* show the reverse reactions.

Principle

Members of the *Enterobacteriaceae* family can be divided into two groups based on the way they metabolize glucose. One group produces large amounts of mixed acids (lactic, formic, succinic, and acetic). When methyl red reagent is added to one of these cultures, a red color is produced owing to the acidic pH. The other group produces predominately neutral end product, acetoin or acetylmethylcarbinol by the butylene glycol pathway. When α-naphthol and 40% potassium hydroxide are added to the broth culture, acetoin, if present, is oxidized to diacetyl in the presence of air and base. α-Naphthol catalyzes a reaction between diacetyl and guanidine components of peptone to produce a pink-red color.

Formulation

Peptone	7 g
Dipotassium phosphate	5 g
Glucose	5 g
Distilled water	1,000 mL
Final pH 6.9	

Preparation and Special Considerations

Mix, heat to boiling, and dispense 1 mL per tube. Autoclave at 121°C for 15 minutes. For methyl red test, broth culture must be incubated for 48 hours. Avoid using really turbid broth. The Voges-Proskauer test was originally designed to be performed after 5 days of incubation at 30°C. By using 0.5 to 1 mL of broth per tube, the test can be done after 18 to 24 hours of incubation at 35°C. Shaking aerates the broth culture and enhances the reaction.

Middlebrook 7H10 and 7H11 Agars

Purpose

The purpose of Middlebrook 7H10 and 7H11 agars is to cultivate *Mycobacterium* species. Isoniazid-resistant strains grow better on these media than on egg-based media, such as Löwenstein-Jensen. The Middlebrook agars are also more chemically defined than Löwenstein-Jensen formulations.

Principle

Middlebrook 7H10 and 7H11 are similar except 7H11 contains casein hydrolysate. Both media contain growth factors, such as amino acids and salts, which encourage recovery of mycobacteria. In addition, both formulations include OADC enrichment, which chemically simulates egg components. Malachite green adds some selectivity.

Formulation

Basal Medium.

Enzymatic hydrolysate of casein	1	g
Ammonium sulfate	0.5	g
Sodium citrate	0.4	g
D-Glutamic acid	0.5	g
Disodium phosphate	1.5	g
Monopotassium phosphate	1.5	g
Ferric ammonium citrate	0.04	g
Magnesium sulfate	0.25	mg
Glycerol	5	mL
Pyridoxine HCl	1	mg
Zinc sulfate	1	mg
Copper sulfate	1	mL
Calcium chloride	0.5	mg
Biotin	0.5	mg
Malachite green	0.25	mg
Agar	15	g
Distilled water	900	mL

Final pH 6.7 to 6.8

OADC Enrichment.

Oleic acid	0.5	g
Bovine albumin, fraction V	50	g
Glucose	20	g
Beef catalase	0.04	g
Sodium chloride	8.5	g
Distilled water	1,000	mL

Final pH 7.0

Preparation and Special Considerations

Prepare basal medium by dissolving powder in distilled water containing 0.5% glycerol. Heat the solution to boiling and distribute 180 mL per flask. Autoclave the flasks at 121°C for 10 minutes; cool to 50°C before adding OADC enrichment, 20 mL per 180 mL basal medium. Pour into plates or dispense into tubes. Medium should be protected from light and stored in plastic wrap at 4°C. Shelf-life is about 2 months. Antibiotics can be added to this basic formulation to prevent overgrowth with bacteria. Mycobacteria selective agar contains cycloheximide, lincomycin HCl, and nalidixic acid. Mitchison 7H11 selective agar is more selective owing to addition of amphotericin B, carbenicillin, polymyxin B, and trimethoprim.

Motility Test Medium

Purpose

The purpose of motility test medium is to determine whether an organism is motile or nonmotile. This test is particularly useful in the identification of

Enterobacteriaceae, in which two genera, *Shigella* and *Klebsiella,* are always nonmotile and certain *Yersinia* species show positive room temperature but no 35°C motility. *Listeria monocytogenes* gives a classic umbrella-type motility, and the non–glucose-fermenting, gram-negative rods can be differentiated in part based on their motility.

Principle

Nonmotile organisms, whick lack flagella, grow only along the stab line, and the surrounding medium remains clear. Motile organisms, which usually possess flagella, move out from the stab line, and the medium appears cloudy. Low agar concentration makes the medium semisolid and permits better detection of motility.

Formulation

Beef extract	3.0 g
Pancreatic hydrolysate of gelatin or peptone	10 g
Sodium chloride	5 g
Agar	4 g
Distilled water	1,000 mL
Final pH 7.3 to 7.4	

Preparation and Special Considerations

Mix powder in distilled water, and heat to boiling. Distribute into tubes; autoclave at 121°C for 15 minutes. Allow to cool as deeps. Use an inoculating needle to stab the medium. Be careful to remove the needle along the initial stab line, and do not stab the medium clear to the tube's bottom. Incubate the inoculated medium at 35°C. Because flagellar protein is not formed as well at higher temperatures, some microbiologists prefer incubation at 18 to 21°C. For *Yersinia,* noting motility reaction at room temperature is particularly useful. Triphenyltetrazolium chloride (TTC) may be added to the basic motility medium to enhance detection of motility. A 1% solution of TTC is prepared and filter sterilized. To 1 L of motility medium, add 5 mL of this solution. If TTC is used, bacteria incorporate colorless TTC and reduce it to red formazan pigment. The medium shows reddening where there is growth. Other media such as SIM (sulfide indole motility) and MIO (motility indole ornithine) can be used to detect motility in addition to other reactions.

Mueller-Hinton Agar

Purpose

Mueller-Hinton agar is a transparent medium, useful for testing susceptibility of organisms to antibiotics. The medium has also been used for testing starch hydrolysis.

Principle

Because Mueller-Hinton agar contains animal infusion, casamino acids, and starch, it supports the growth of most organisms. In addition, sheep blood may be added to the basic formulation to perform susceptibility testing on streptococci. The addition of heated or chocolatized sheep blood to Mueller-Hinton agar makes possible the testing of fastidious organisms such as *Haemophilus* and *Neisseria*. Starch is included in the medium for two reasons. It may protect the organisms against toxic substances. Also, it serves as an energy source. Calcium and magnesium concentrations are critical in the testing of *Pseudomonas* isolates with aminoglycoside antibiotics. Usually Mueller-Hinton agar contains sufficient amounts of calcium and magnesium, but it may be necessary to add these substances to Mueller-Hinton broth.

Formulation

Beef extract	300	g
Casamino acids (acid hydrolysate of casein)	17.5	g
Starch, soluble	1.5	g
Agar	17	g
Distilled water	1,000	mL
Final pH 7.4		

Preparation and Special Considerations

Mix powder in distilled water; heat to boiling. Autoclave at 116 to 121°C for 15 minutes. Pour plates with optimal depth of 4 mm. Cool the plates with lids ajar to prevent excess moisture from forming on the agar's surface. Store in sealed plastic bags in the refrigerator. For Mueller-Hinton agar with sheep blood, cool the basal medium to 45 to 50°C and add 50 to 100 mL of defibrinated sheep blood. After gentle mixing, pour quickly into plates. For Mueller-Hinton chocolate agar, add a similar volume of sheep blood to basal medium, but heat the mixture at 80°C for 15 minutes or until the medium changes to brown color. This procedure releases NAD and hemoglobin and destroys heat-labile inhibitors. Mueller-Hinton broth is similar in formulation to Mueller-Hinton agar except it lacks agar. Some broth formulations include a "cation" supplement of 0.1% glucose, 2.0% Isovitalex, 25 mg Mg^{2+}, and 50 mg Ca^{2+} per liter.

New York City Medium

Purpose

The purpose of New York City medium is to isolate *Neisseria gonorrhoeae* and *Neisseria meningitidis* from specimens containing mixed normal flora.

Principle

New York City medium contains hemoglobin, yeast dialysate, and horse plasma, making it highly enriched to support the growth of *Neisseria gonorrhoeae* and *Neisseria meningitidis.* Selectivity for these two organisms is accomplished by four antibiotics that inhibit normal flora. Vancomycin prevents the growth of gram-positive bacteria; colistin inhibits gram-negative rods; amphotericin B prevents growth of yeast and molds. Trimethoprim has been included to prevent swarming of *Proteus* species. Cornstarch, another component, absorbs toxic substances that could otherwise inhibit the growth of these *Neisseria* species.

Formulation

Basal medium (melted and cooled to 55°C, see next)	120 mL
3% Hemoglobin solution (see next)	200 mL
50% Glucose solution (see next)	10 mL
Yeast dialysate (see next)	25 mL
Antibiotic mixture (see next)	5 mL

Preparation of solutions used in formulation is as follows:

1. Agar solution

   Agar   20 g
   Distilled water   400 mL
   Heat to boiling until agar is melted.
2. Cornstarch solution

   Cornstarch   1 g
   Distilled water   40 mL
   Mix on a magnetic stirring plate, and heat to boiling until solution appears homogeneous.
3. Proteose peptone solution

   Proteose peptone no. 3   15 g
   Dipotassium phosphate   4 g
   Monopotassium phosphate   1 g
   Sodium chloride   5 g
   Distilled water   200 mL
   Using a magnetic stirrer, heat the solution to boiling. Final pH should be 7.1 ± 0.1.

To prepare basal medium, combine solutions 1, 2, and 3. Mix thoroughly, and autoclave at 121°C for 15 minutes. Cool and store in refrigerator until needed.

Additives

1. 3% Hemoglobin solution

   Horse or human red blood cells   6 mL
   Sterile distilled water   200 mL
   In the presence of distilled water, red blood cells lyse to form a hemoglobin solution. Store solution in refrigerator until needed.
2. 50% Glucose solution

   Glucose   5 g
   Distilled water   10 mL

Sterilize in autoclave at 110°C for 10 minutes or by filter (0.45 μm pore size). Store solution in refrigerator until needed.

3. Citrated horse plasma

Sodium chloride   4.8 g
Sodium citrate   90 g
Distilled water   add to 600 mL total volume

Sterilize solution at 115°C for 10 minutes. Draw horse blood to 6 L to form a 10% final concentration of citrate.

4. Antibiotic mixture

Vancomycin   2 μg/mL
Colistin   5.5 μg/mL
Amphotericin B   1.2 μg/mL
Trimethoprim lactate 3 μg/mL

Mix solutions together. Freeze at -20°C until ready to use.

5. Yeast dialysate

Bakers' yeast   908 g
Distilled water   2,500 mL

Combine yeast and water to make a smooth paste. Autoclave at 121°C for 10 minutes. Cool, and place mixture into dialysis tubing. Dialyze against 2 L of cold water. Collect the dialysate, and dispense in aliquots. Autoclave at 121°C for 15 minutes. Store in the freezer indefinitely.

Preparation and Special Considerations

To prepare medium, melt and cool basal medium to 50 to 55°C. Add the other solutions in amounts indicated. Pour into plates and allow to solidify. Store in plastic bags in the refrigerator. Shelf-life is 2 to 2.5 months. Note that the hemoglobin solution is optional. If this solution is omitted, an additional 200 mL of distilled water should be added to the basal medium prior to autoclaving. When using New York City medium for recovery of *N. gonorrhoeae* and *N. meningitidis,* the microbiologist should incubate plates under increased carbon dioxide for several days. Also, a nonselective agar, such as chocolate agar, should be included because 5% of gonococci are inhibited by the antibiotics, particularly vancomycin, found in this medium.

Nitrate Reduction Broth

Purpose

The purpose of nitrate reduction broth is to determine if an organism can reduce nitrate to nitrite or to gaseous products such as nitrogem. The test is useful in the recognition of *Enterobacteriaceae,* most of which can reduce nitrate to nitrite; non–glucose-fermenting, gram-negative rods, and *Moraxella catarrhalis.*

Principle

The nitrate test is performed in two parts. Sulfanilic acid and α-naphthylamine reagents are added first. If nitrate has been reduced to nitrite, nitrite reacts with these reagents to form a red diazonium dye, p-sulfobenzene-azo-naphthylamine. If there is no color change, zinc dust is added. Zinc reduces the remaining nitrate to nitrite to form a red color. If nitrate was reduced all the way to nitrogen gas, however, no color change occurs.

Formulation

Beef extract (or tryptone 5 g)	5 g
Neopeptone or pancreatic hydrolysate of gelatin	5 g
Potassium nitrate	1 g
Distilled water	1,000 mL
Final pH 7.0	

Preparation and Special Considerations

Some formulations include glucose (0.1 g). Before adding potassium nitrate and glucose, heat to boiling, and adjust the pH to 7.3 to 7.4. Aliquot into screw-cap tubes, and place a Durham tube into each. Autoclave the medium at 121°C for 15 minutes. When using this medium, inoculate broth culture for 24 to 48 hours before testing. Observe the Durham tube for presence of gas bubbles. Add 1 mL of sulfanilic acid reagent and 1 mL of α-naphthylamine reagent. Interpret the results immediately because color fades quickly. If it is necessary to add zinc, avoid using large amounts. Too much zinc can result in formation of hydrogen gas, which can cause reduction and decrease the color reaction. Medium may need to be supplemented with serum and incubated up to 5 days when testing *Neisseria*. Because α-naphthylamine is carcinogenic, it is preferable to substitute N,N-dimethyl-α-naphthylamine.

Nutrient Agar

Purpose

Nutrient agar has been used to distinguish between the nonfastidious, less pathogenic *Neisseria* species and pathogenic *Neisseria,* such as *N. gonorrhoeae* and *N. meningitidis.* The less fastidious *Neisseria* grow on nutrient agar, whereas the more pathogenic species do not. Nutrient agar has also been used for maintenance of stock cultures.

Principle

Nutrient agar contains minimal nutrients and an especially low concentration of protein. Growth of an isolate on this medium means that it is not fastidious and does not require special supplements.

Formulation

Pancreatic hydrolysate of gelatin (or peptone)	5 g
Beef extract	3 g

Agar	15 g
Distilled water	1,000 mL
Final pH 6.8	

Preparation and Special Considerations

Mix ingredients together and heat to boiling. Dispense into tubes if desired. Autoclave at 121°C for 15 minutes. Pour into Petri dishes and cool.

Oxidative-Fermentative Medium (Hugh and Leifson Formulation)

Purpose

Oxidative-fermentative medium is useful in determining an organism's type of carbohydrate utilization—oxidative, fermentative, or inert. This medium is important in the identification of non–glucose-fermenting, gram-negative rods.

Principle

Three modifications over traditional media for detection of fermentation make this medium useful for testing nonfermenting gram-negative rods. A low concentration of peptone prevents formation of alkaline products that may neutralize the small quantities of acid produced through oxidation. The high concentration of carbohydrate increases the potential amount of acid that can be formed. The lower concentration of agar makes the medium semisolid. This permits acid formed on the surface to diffuse throughout the medium. Bromthymol blue serves as the pH indicator for acid detection.

Formulation

Basal medium.

Peptone or tryptone	2	g
Sodium chloride	5	g
Bromthymol blue	0.03	g
Agar	3	g (2.5 g in some formulations)
Dipotassium phosphate	0.3	g
Distilled water	1,000	mL
Final pH 7.1		

Additives.

10% Carbohydrate solutions

Carbohydrate (glucose, lactose, sucrose, or other)	2 g
Distilled water	20 mL

After mixing the carbohydrate in water and stirring until dissolved, use a filter (0.2 μg/mL) to sterilize.

Preparation and Special Considerations

Heat the basal medium to boiling to dissolve powder. Autoclave at 121°C for 15 minutes; cool to 55°C. For every 200 mL of medium, aseptically add 20 mL of sterilized carbohydrate solution. This makes a 1% final concentration of carbohydrate. Aliquot into tubes and allow to cool as deeps. The classic method for using this medium involves the stabbing of two tubes with the organism. The medium in one tube is covered with vaspar (a mixture of petrolatum and paraffin) or melted paraffin. Sterile mineral oil has been used for this purpose, but it is not recommended because it does not block out oxygen as well. Results are interpreted after 35°C incubation. Several days of incubation may be required owing to slower growth of some nonfermenting gram-negative rods. Color change to yellow in both tubes means that the organism is fermentative (can produce acid in absence of oxygen). Color change to yellow in uncovered tube only means that the organism is oxidative (requires oxygen to use the carbohydrate). If neither tube changes in color or covered tube shows no change while uncovered tube turns blue, the organism cannot use the carbohydrate oxidatively or fermentatively and is considered inert. A one-tube modification of this test has been described. One tube is stabbed and not covered. Color change to yellow near top of medium only indicates oxidative use of glucose. If the entire tube changes to yellow, fermentation is suggested. Because the medium is semisolid, motility may be observed in this medium. *Note:* Sometimes oxidative-fermentative medium is used for differentiating staphylococci (fermentative) from micrococci (oxidative). This testing requires a different formulation.

Peptone-Yeast Extract-Glucose Broth (PYG)

Purpose

Peptone-yeast extract-glucose broth is useful for culturing anaerobes. PYG broth culture of an anaerobic isolate may be used in gas liquid chromatography procedures that detect metabolic end products.

Principle

PYG broth contains several nutrients and supplements that encourage the growth of anaerobes. These enrichments include vitamin K (required for pigment-producing *Prevotella* and *Porphyromonas*), yeast extract, hemin, and glucose. Cysteine helps to keep the medium more reduced and anaerobic. Resazurin serves as an anaerobic indicator. Pink color means that oxygen is present.

Formulation

Peptone	5 g
Trypticase	5 g

Yeast extract	10	g
D-Glucose	10	g
Salt solution	40	mL
Resazurin solution	4	mL
Hemin solution	10	mL
Vitamin K	0.2	mL
Cysteine hydrochloride	0.5	g
Distilled water	1,000	mL

Final pH 7.2

Solutions required for preparation are as follows:

1. Salt solution

Calcium chloride	0.2	g
Magnesium sulfate	0.2	g
Potassium monohydrogen phosphate	1	g
Potassium dihydrogen phosphate	1	g
Sodium bicarbonate	10	g
Sodium chloride	2	g

First mix the calcium chloride and magnesium sulfate in 200 mL of distilled water. Once these components are dissolved, add an additional 500 mL of water and the other salts. Continue mixing until all salts are dissolved and add an additional 200 mL of water. Store in refrigerator.

2. Resazurin solution

Resazurin	25 mg
Water, distilled	100 mL

Dissolve resazurin in water. Store the solution at room temperature.

Preparation and Special Considerations

Mix all ingredients except the vitamin K, hemin, and cysteine. After heating to boiling, cool to 50°C, and add these last three components. Aliquot the medium into tubes; autoclave at 115°C for 15 minutes. *Note:* One formulation has 20 g of peptone in place of peptone/trypticase of the above-listed recipe and lacks hemin and vitamin K. Some formulations of the salt solution do not include sodium bicarbonate and sodium chloride. This medium should be prereduced before it is used. Mixing of this tubed medium might expose deeper parts of medium to oxygen and prevent anaerobic growth.

Phenylalanine Deaminase Agar (PAD)

Purpose

Phenylalanine deaminase agar is used to detect the organism's ability to deaminate or remove the amino group from phenylalanine. A positive reaction is most useful for distinguishing *Proteus, Providencia,* and *Morganella* from other members of the family *Enterobacteriaceae.* This test can also be used to distinguish *Moraxella phenylpyruvica* (+) from other *Moraxella.*

Principle

Phenylalanine deaminase agar includes phenylalanine, the amino acid to be deaminated; yeast extract, a nitrogen and carbon source; various salts; and agar, a solidifying agent. Protein hydrolysates and meat extracts are not included because these substances contain a variable amount of phenylalanine. If an organism produces phenylalanine deaminase, it can convert phenylalanine to the α-keto acid called phenylpyruvic acid. This acid reacts with the added ferric chloride reagent to form a dark green complex. The immediate appearance of a dark green slant on addition of ferric chloride reagent is a positive reaction; no color change on addition of reagent is a negative reaction.

Formulation

DL-Phenylalanine	2 g
Yeast extract	3 g
Sodium chloride	5 g
Sodium phosphate	1 g
Agar	12 g
Distilled water	1,000 mL
Final pH 7.3	

Preparation and Special Considerations

Mix powder in water, and heat to boiling. Dispense medium into tubes. Autoclave at 121°C for 10 minutes. Cool in a slanted position. Add several drops of ferric chloride reagent to slant of 24- to 48-hour culture. Rotate the tube to insure that reagent makes as much contact with culture as possible. A positive reaction occurs within 1 to 5 minutes and should be interpreted as soon as possible because the color tends to fade quickly.

Phenylethyl Alcohol Agar (PEA)

Purpose

Phenylethyl alcohol agar isolates gram-positive cocci such as staphylococci and streptococci from specimens having mixed flora. The anaerobic formulation of this medium selects for gram-negative and gram-positive nonsporulating anaerobes, while inhibiting the facultatively anaerobic gram-negative rods and other anaerobes.

Principle

PEA is similar to sheep blood agar except it contains phenylethyl alcohol. This component inhibits facultative gram-negative rods, especially swarming *Proteus,* but permits the growth of gram-positive cocci.

Formulation

Tryptose (alternative: pancreatic digest of casein or casein peptone—15 g)	10	g
Beef extract (alternative: papaic digest of soy meal or soy peptone—5 g)	3	g
Sodium chloride	5	g
Phenylethyl alcohol (phenylethanol)	2.5	g
Agar	15	g
Distilled water	1,000	mL
Final pH 7.3 ± 0.2		

Preparation and Special Considerations

Mix powder in distilled water, and heat to boiling to dissolve. Avoid over-heating because this can inactivate the phenylethyl alcohol. Autoclave the medium at 121°C for 15 minutes. Cool to 50°C, and add 50 mL of defibrinated sheep blood. Pour into plates. Phenylethyl alcohol is volatile, and plates should be tightly sealed in plastic bags and stored in the refrigerator. Hemolytic reactions are not dependable on this medium owing to the action of phenylethyl alcohol on cell membranes. Gram-negative rods may grow on PEA, but colonies are smaller than usual and can be readily differentiated from those of gram-positive rods. *Pseudomonas aeruginosa* is not inhibited by this medium. Some gram-positive cocci may require more than 24 hours of incubation to grow well on PEA. An anaerobic formulation can be achieved by adding 2.5 g of phenylethyl alcohol to 1 L of CDC anaerobic agar before autoclaving or by supplementing the above-listed formulation with vitamin K (10 μg/mL) as well as sheep blood after sterilization of basal medium.

Pseudocel (Cetrimide) Agar

Purpose

Pseudocel or cetrimide agar is used to select for *P. aeruginosa* in specimens with mixed flora. Also, because it inhibits other *Pseudomonas* species (except *Pseudomonas fluorescens*) and closely related organisms, this test can be useful in the differentiation of non–glucose-fermenting, gram-negative rods.

Principle

This medium contains cetrimide, also called cetyl trimethyl ammonium bromide or hexadecyltrimethylammonium bromide. Produced from bromine, cetrimide is highly inhibitory and has been used as an antiseptic. If the organism can tolerate cetrimide, it grows on the medium. Magnesium chloride and potassium sulfate stimulate the production of pyocyanin, the green pigment characteristically produced by *P. aeruginosa*.

Formulation

Pancreatic digest of gelatin or peptone	20	g
Magnesium chloride	1.4	g
Potassium sulfate	10	g
Agar, dried	13.6	g
Cetrimide	0.3	g
Distilled water	1,000	mL
Final pH 7.2		

Preparation and Special Considerations

Mix ingredients in water; add 10 mL of glycerol. Heat and boil for 1 minute. Distribute into tubes before autoclaving, or pour into plates following autoclaving. Autoclave at 118 to 121°C for 15 minutes. Lots of cetrimide may differ. Therefore, careful quality control with known strains is critical in establishing that the medium works.

Salmonella-Shigella Agar (SS)

Purpose

Salmonella-Shigella agar is used to select for *Salmonella* and some strains of *Shigella* from stool specimens. SS agar is also differential in that these organisms produce characteristic colonies on the medium.

Principle

SS agar contains bile salts, sodium citrate, and brilliant green, which inhibit the growth of gram-positive rods and many lactose-fermenting gram-negative rods normally found in feces. Lactose serves as the sole carbohydrate source in the medium; neutral red serves as a pH indicator. If an organism grows on the medium and ferments lactose, it produces acid and changes the indicator to pink-red. Sodium thiosulfate acts as a source of sulfur for the production of hydrogen sulfide. If hydrogen sulfide is produced, it reacts with ferric chloride present in the medium to form a black precipitate in the center of the colony.

Formulation

Beef extract	5	g
Peptone	5	g
Lactose	10	g
Bile salts	8.5	g
Sodium citrate	8.5	g
Sodium thiosulfate	8.5	g

Ferric citrate	1	g
Agar	13.5	g
Brilliant green	0.33	g
Neutral red	0.025	g
Distilled water	1,000	mL

Final pH 7.4

Preparation and Special Considerations

Mix powder in water and dissolve by boiling briefly. Do not autoclave this medium. Cool to 50°C, and pour into plates. Allow surface of plates to dry before placing in plastic bags and storing in refrigerator. A heavy inoculum of stool can be planted on SS agar because the formulation is so inhibitory. Strains of *Shigella* may not grow on SS agar, however, and this medium should not be used as the sole primary plating medium when *Shigella* is the potential isolate. *Shigella* colonies appear colorless on SS agar because these organisms do not ferment lactose or produce hydrogen sulfide. *Salmonella* produces colorless colonies with a black center because these organisms usually make hydrogen sulfide but do not ferment lactose. Pink-to-red colonies indicate that the organism ferments lactose; if there is a black center, it also produces hydrogen sulfide. If *Proteus* grows on this medium, swarming is inhibited.

Selenite F Broth

Purpose

Selenite F broth is an enrichment broth used for the recovery of low numbers of *Salmonella* and some strains of *Shigella* from stool and other specimens containing large amounts of mixed bacteria.

Principle

The sodium selenite present in this medium inhibits the growth of many gram-negative rods and enterococci but permits recovery of *Salmonella* species and some *Shigella* species. Selenite is most effective at a neutral pH. Reduction of selenite during growth of bacteria produces alkaline products, so lactose is also included in this medium. Lactose fermenters produce acid, which neutralizes these alkaline products and returns the medium to a neutral pH.

Formulation

Peptone	5 g
Lactose	4 g
Sodium selenite	4 g
Sodium phosphate	10 g

Distilled water   1,000 mL
Final pH 7.0

Preparation and Special Considerations

Dissolve powder in distilled water, heat to boiling, and dispense into tubes. Because this medium is most effective under anaerobic conditions, try to have at least a 2-inch depth in the tube. To sterilize, place tubes in autoclave and expose to 30 minutes of flowing steam. Do not autoclave. Overheating causes formation of a precipitate that makes the medium unusable. When using selenite broth, the microbiologist should subculture the broth to enteric media after it has incubated 8 to 12 hours. Beyond this time frame, overgrowth with normal flora is likely.

Sodium Chloride Broth, 6.5%

Purpose

Sodium chloride broth is useful in the differentiation of streptococci, particularly those producing α and nonhemolytic colonies. Primarily, it distinguishes *Enterococcus* species (+) from group D streptococci (−), both of which produce a positive bile esculin agar slant. Also, viridans streptococci cannot grow in this medium.

Principle

Sodium chloride broth is prepared from heart infusion broth, a general purpose medium, which already contains 0.5% sodium chloride. By adding 6% sodium chloride to this medium, the salt concentration becomes 6.5%. Sodium chloride broth also contains glucose as a carbohydrate source and bromcresol purple, a pH indicator. If the organism can tolerate this high concentration of salt, it grows in the medium and produces cloudiness. Fermentation of glucose produces acid and may cause the medium to turn yellow.

Formulation

Heart infusion broth   1,000 mL
Sodium chloride   60 g
Bromcresol purple indicator   1 mL
Glucose   1 g
Final pH 7.4

Additives.

1. Heart infusion broth
   Infusion from beef heart muscle   375 g

Tryptose or thiotone peptic digest of animal tissue	10 g
Sodium chloride	5.0 g
Distilled water	1,000 mL

2. Bromcresol purple indicator

| Bromcresol purple | 1.6 g |
| 95% ethanol | 100 mL |

Preparation and Special Considerations

Mix components and heat to boiling to dissolve. Dispense into tubes. Autoclave at 121°C for 15 minutes. Store in refrigerator. Some formulations omit indicator and glucose. To use medium, inoculate several colonies into broth, and incubate culture overnight at 35°C. Any growth in the broth is considered positive even if the indicator does not change color. To avoid false-negative results, gently mix broth before interpretation. Inoculating the broth too heavily may give a false-positive result. Organisms other than enterococci can produce positive results, i.e., group B streptococci and aerococci.

SP-4 Broth/Agar

Purpose

SP-4 broth and SP-4 agar serve as primary isolation media for *Mycoplasma* species.

Principle

SP-4 media contain yeast products that serve as growth factors for *Mycoplasma* and supply preformed nucleic acid. Fetal bovine serum supplies the cholesterol necessary for stabilizing these organisms because they lack cell walls. Various antibiotics inhibit normal flora, which may be present in the specimen. Penicillin is included to prevent growth of gram-positive bacteria, amphotericin B inhibits fungi, and polymyxin B inhibits gram-negative rods. Biphasic media provide both microaerophilic and moist conditions, which some *Mycoplasma* species prefer.

Formulation

Basal medium, cooled to 56°C	625 mL
CMRL 1066 tissue culture medium with glutamate	50 mL
Yeast dialysate	35 mL
Yeastolate, 2%	100 mL
Fetal bovine serum (heat-inactivated at 56°C for 30 minutes)	170 mL
Penicillin G (or ampicillin 1 mg/mL)	1,000,000 U

Amphotericin B	0.5 g
Polymyxin B	500,000 U

Additives.

1. Basal medium

Mycoplasma broth base	3.5 g
Tryptone or pancreatic digest of casein	10 g
Bacto-Peptone or proteose pancreatic digest of gelatin (5.3 g)	5 g
Glucose, 50%	10 mL
Distilled water	615.5 mL
Final pH 7.5	

2. 50% glucose solution

D-Glucose	10 g
Distilled water	20 mL

Mix and sterilize by membrane filtration.

Preparation and Special Considerations

Prepare basal medium by mixing components and heating just to boiling. Adjust pH to 7.5. Autoclave at 121°C for 15 minutes. Cool to 56°C before adding supplements. Yeast dialysate can be prepared in the same manner as for New York City medium. Many of these components are available from various commercial companies. If SP-4 agar is desired, add 8.5 g of Nobel agar to the basal medium. Biphasic medium may be prepared by dispensing 1 mL of SP-4 agar into screw-cap vials and allowing this to harden into slants. Overlay with 2 ml SP-4 broth. Seal tightly and store in the freezer at −20°C.

SP-4—Arginine, Glucose, and Urea Broths

Purpose

SP-4 broths are useful in the identification of *Mycoplasma* and *Ureaplasma*.

Principle

Yeast products included in SP-4 broth supply nutrients required for growth of *Mycoplasma* and *Ureaplasma*. Fetal bovine serum contains cholesterol, which helps stabilize these organisms because they lack cell walls. Penicillin prevents growth of gram-positive cocci but does not affect these organisms because they do not possess cell walls. Phenol red serves as a pH indicator. In SP-4 arginine broth, utilization of arginine results in alkaline products and color change to red. This reaction characterizes *Mycoplasma hominis*. In SP-4 urea broth, removal of amino group from urea, characteristic of *Ureaplasma*, causes formation of ammonia and a similar color change to red. SP-4 glucose broth detects glucose fermentation. Acid is produced, which lowers medium pH and changes its color to yellow. This reaction typifies *Mycoplasma pneumoniae* as well as a few other *Mycoplasma* sp.

Formulation

Basal medium, cooled to 50°C	61.5 mL
Sterile supplements	38.5 mL
50% urea	0.1 mL
or	
50% glucose	1 mL
or	
50% arginine	1 mL
Final pH 7.4	

Basal Medium.

Mycoplasma broth base	3.5 g
Tryptone or pancreatic digest of casein	10 g
Proteose pancreatic digest of gelatin	5.3 g
Distilled water	615 mL
Final pH 7.5	

Sterile Supplements.

CMRL 1066 tissue culture medium with glutamate	50 mL
Yeast dialysate	35 mL
Yeastolate, 2%	100 mL
Fetal bovine serum (heat-inactivated at 56°C for 60 minutes)	170 mL
Penicillin G, 100,000 units/mL	10 mL
Phenol red, 0.1%	20 mL

Additives.

1. 50% urea solution

Urea	5 g
Distilled water	10 g

   Mix and filter sterilize. Store at −20°C.
2. 50% glucose solution

D-Glucose	10 g
Distilled water	20 mL

   Mix and sterilize by membrane filtration. Store at −20°C.
3. 50% arginine solution

L-Arginine	10 g
Distilled water	20 mL

   Mix and sterilize by membrane filtration. Store at −20°C.

Preparation and Special Considerations

Mix components of basal medium, heat to boiling, and adjust pH to 7.5. Autoclave at 121°C for 15 minutes. Prepare sterile supplements mixture and the appropriate additives. Cool basal medium to 50°C before combining.

Tetrathionate Broth

Purpose

Tetrathionate broth is an enrichment medium used for recovery of low numbers of *Salmonella* species from stool specimens.

Principle

Bile salt in conjunction with thiosulfate and added iodine-iodide solution inhibits the growth of gram-positive organisms and most gram-negative rods except *Salmonella*. Some formulations also include brilliant green or crystal violet, which increases the inhibitory nature of the medium.

Formulation

Basal medium   1,000 mL
Iodine solution   20 mL
Final pH 7.0

Basal Medium.

Proteose peptone (pancreatic digest of casein and peptic digest of animal tissue)	5 g
Bile salts	1 g
Calcium carbonate	10 g
Sodium thiosulfate	30 g
Distilled water	1,000 mL

Iodine Solution.

Iodine	6 g
Potassium iodide	5 g
Distilled water	20 mL

Preparation and Special Considerations

Tetrathionate basal medium is prepared by mixing components and heating to boiling. Cool medium to 45°C, and add the iodine solution. Do not autoclave and do not heat the medium after addition of the iodine solution. Distribute 10 mL per tube. The medium must be used within 24 hours of preparation. Because the basal medium may be stored in the refrigerator indefinitely, some microbiologists prefer to dispense basal medium 10 mL per tube. Just before use, 0.2 mL of iodine solution can be added to each tube. Heavy inoculum of stool can be added to the broth. After 12 to 24 hours of incubation at 35°C, the broth should be subcultured to enteric media to prevent overgrowth with normal flora. This medium inhibits most *Shigella* and should not be used for recovering *Salmonella typhi.*

Thayer-Martin, Modified Agar

Purpose

Modified Thayer-Martin agar is an enriched, selective medium used for recovering *N. gonorrhoeae* and *N. meningitidis* from specimens with mixed flora.

Principle

Modified Thayer-Martin agar is highly enriched to support the growth of the more fastidious *Neisseria* species. Added growth factors include hemoglobin, vitamins, cocarboxylase, diphosphopyridine nucleotide, and glutamine. Cornstarch is included to absorb any inhibitory substances that might be present. The modified formulation contains more agar, which may help to prevent swarming of *Proteus*. Modified Thayer-Martin agar contains several antibiotics that together inhibit normal flora and prevent the growth of most other organisms. Vancomycin inhibits gram-positive cocci. Colistin inhibits gram-negative rods, whereas trimethoprim prevents *Proteus* from swarming. Nystatin prevents the growth of fungi.

Formulation

GC agar base, double strength	500 mL
2% Hemoglobin solution	500 mL
Growth supplements (Isovitalex—BBL or Bacto-Supplement B—Difco)	10 mL
Antimicrobic solution (CNVT—Difco)	10 mL
Final pH 7.2	

Preparation of component solutions is as follows:

1. GC agar base, double strength

Pancreatic digest of casein	7.5 g
Pancreatic digest of animal tissue (15 g of peptone may be substituted for both of above)	7.5 g
Cornstarch	1 g
Dipotassium phosphate	4 g
Monopotassium phosphate	1 g
Sodium chloride	5 g
Agar	10 g
Distilled water	500 mL

Additions to GC agar base include:

Agar	2 g
D-Glucose	5 g

2. 2% hemoglobin solution

Hemoglobin	10 g
Distilled water	500 mL

3. Growth supplements, i.e., Isovitalex (commercially available)

Vitamin B_{12}	0.01	g
L-Glutamine	10	g
Adenine	1	g
Guanine hydrochloride	0.03	g
p-Aminobenzoic acid	0.013	g
L-Cystine	1.1	g
Glucose	100	g
Diphosphopyridine nucleotide	0.25	g
Cocarboxylase	0.1	g
Ferric nitrate	0.02	g
Thiamine hydrochloride	0.003	g
Cysteine hydrochloride	25.9	g
Distilled water	1,000	mL

4. Antimicrobic solution

Vancomycin	3,000	μg
Colistin sulfate	7,500	μg
Nystatin	12,500	units
Trimethoprim lactate	5,000	μg
Distilled water	10	mL

Preparation and Special Considerations

Prepare double-strength GC base by dissolving powder in 500 mL of distilled water. Add 2 g of agar and 5 g of glucose to this solution, heat to boiling, and autoclave at 121°C for 15 minutes. Prepare hemoglobin solution by dissolving hemoglobin in water and heating to boiling. Autoclave at 121°C for 15 minutes. Cool both solutions to 50°C, and maintain temperature by placing them in a water bath. Combine these solutions, and add antibiotics and growth supplements. Pour into plates. Wrap plates in plastic and store in refrigerator.

Five percent, chocolatized, defibrinated sheep blood may be substituted for the hemoglobin solution. The original Thayer-Martin formulation lacked additional agar and glucose as well as the trimethoprim and is, therefore, not as effective at inhibiting swarming *Proteus*. The Martin-Lewis formulation substitutes anisomycin, 20 μg/mL, for nystatin as the antifungal agent. In addition, vancomycin concentration of 4 μg/mL is higher than in the modified Thayer-Martin formulation.

When using modified Thayer-Martin plates, the microbiologist should incubate them in a carbon dioxide incubator or candle jar for several days. Because some strains of *N. gonorrhoeae* may be inhibited by vancomycin, a chocolate plate should also be planted.

Thioglycolate Broth, Basal and Enriched

Purpose

Thioglycolate broth is an all-purpose medium that can be used to isolate a wide range of bacteria. It is often employed as a back-up broth that is inoculated along with culture plates. In this case, it helps detect those organisms that were present in low numbers or anaerobes in the original specimen. When glucose is omitted, thioglycolate broth can be used in fermentation studies of anaerobes.

Principle

Thioglycolate, cystine, and sodium sulfite act as reducing agents in this medium, whereas the low concentration of agar prevents downward diffusion of oxygen. Various supplements can be added to support the growth of more fastidious organisms.

Formulation

Pancreatic digest of casein	17	g
Papaic digest of soy meal	3	g
Glucose	6	g
Sodium chloride	2.5	g
Sodium thioglycollate	0.5	g
L-Cystine	0.25	g
Sodium sulfite	0.1	g
Agar	0.7	g
Distilled water	1,000	mL

Preparation and Special Considerations

Mix components in distilled water and heat to boiling. Dispense into tubes; autoclave at 121°C for 15 minutes.

Various supplements can be added to the basic formulation, including hemin (5 μg/mL), vitamin K (0.1 μg/mL), and sodium bicarbonate (1 mg/mL), which can be autoclaved in medium. Supplements that must be added after autoclaving include rabbit or horse serum (10% vol/vol) and Fildes enrichment (5% vol/vol). These are given as final concentrations in the medium.

Thioglycolate broth should be stored at room temperature and boiled and cooled before use. When used as a back-up broth, the medium is incubated at 35°C for 3 to 7 days and examined for turbidity. Gram stains of broth are compared with growth obtained on primary culture plates. If something different appears to be growing in the broth, subcultures should be done.

Thiosulfate-Citrate-Bile Salts-Sucrose Agar (TCBS)

Purpose

Thiosulfate-citrate-bile salts-sucrose agar is a selective medium used to isolate *Vibrio* species from stool specimens having mixed flora. TCBS is also differential in that *Vibrio* species produce characteristic colonies.

Principle

Vibrio species grow poorly on media designed for isolation of *Salmonella* and *Shigella* but produce colorless colonies on MacConkey. TCBS includes sodium citrate, sodium thiosulfate, and oxgall (10% solution equivalent to full-strength bile), which together inhibit many gram-positive cocci and gram-negative rods normally present in stool specimens. In addition, the high pH of TCBS agar encourages the growth of *Vibrio*, while inhibiting other organisms. Different types of colonies are produced by different species of *Vibrio* owing to the presence of sucrose as a fermentable carbohydrate and bromthymol blue as a pH indicator. For example, *Vibrio cholerae* and *Vibrio alginolyticus* produce yellow colonies because they can ferment sucrose, whereas *Vibrio parahaemolyticus* and *Vibrio vulnificus* usually produce blue-green colonies owing to lack of sucrose fermentation. Organisms that can produce hydrogen sulfide from sodium thiosulfate have black centers as a result of reaction of this gas with ferric citrate. Vibrios do not produce hydrogen sulfide.

Formulation

Yeast extract	5	g
Proteose peptone no. 3 (pancreatic digest of casein and peptic digest of animal tissue)	10	g
Sodium citrate	10	g
Sodium thiosulfate	10	g
Oxgall	8	g
Sucrose	20	g
Ferric citrate	1	g
Bromthymol blue	0.04	g
Agar	15	g
Distilled water	1,000	mL
Final pH 8.6 ± 0.2		

Preparation and Special Considerations

Mix components in distilled water and heat to boiling. Cool to 50°C, and pour into plates. Autoclaving this medium is not recommended. Plates may be stored in the refrigerator for 6 to 8 weeks.

Some formulations include a second pH indicator, thymol blue, at a concentration of 0.04 g/L. Oxgall (5 g/L) and sodium cholate (3 g/L) or bile salts (8 g/L) may be used in place of oxgall alone.

When using TCBS agar, the microbiologist should use a heavy inoculum because *Vibrio* species die off quickly and this medium is inhibitory. Fresh specimen is best because these organisms are sensitive to drying out, sunlight, and acid pH. If there must be a delay in planting, use Cary-Blair semisolid transport medium rather than buffered glycerol transport medium. Plates should be incubated at 35°C for 18 to 24 hours and up to 48 hours. Growth off TCBS is not acceptable for performing oxidase test. Occasional strains of *V. cholerae* may produce blue-green colonies on this medium as a result of delayed sucrose fermentation. Some vibrios do not grow well on this medium. Also, other organisms such as *Pseudomonas, Plesiomonas,* and *Aeromonas* can grow on TCBS and usually produce blue colonies and must be distinguished from vibrios.

Tinsdale Agar

Purpose

Tinsdale agar is a selective differential medium useful in isolating and identifying *C. diphtheriae* from specimens containing mixed flora.

Principle

Tinsdale agar contains a high concentration of potassium tellurite, which inhibits the growth of most normal flora organisms but permits *Corynebacterium* species, especially *C. diphtheriae,* to grow. All *Corynebacterium* species growing on the medium produce gray-to-black colonies owing to the reduction of tellurite to tellurium. In addition, *C. diphtheriae* colonies are surrounded by a brown halo. This brown halo is thought to be produced from tellurite interacting with hydrogen sulfide produced by the organism from cystine and thiosulfate.

Formulation

Basal medium, cooled to 50°C	1,000	mL
Sterile bovine serum	100	mL
Potassium tellurite, 1%, in water, sterile	30	mL

Preparation of basal medium is as follows:

Thiotone peptone (peptic digest of animal tissues)	20	g
Sodium chloride	5	g
L-Cystine	0.24	g
Sodium thiosulfate	0.43	g
Agar	14	g
Distilled water	1,000	mL
Final pH 7.4		

Preparation and Special Considerations

Prepare the basal medium by mixing components with water and heating to boiling. Autoclave at 121°C for 15 minutes. Cool the medium to 50°C, and aseptically add tellurite solution and bovine serum. Pour into plates, and store in refrigerator. Plates have a shelf-life of 4 days. The autoclaved basal medium, however, can be stored indefinitely; tellurite and serum can be added just before use.

When using Tinsdale agar, the microbiologist should streak plates for isolation and stab the medium in several areas. Sometimes browning occurs in these stabbed areas before it can be seen around colonies. Plates should be incubated at 35°C for 24 to 48 hours in ambient air. Increased carbon dioxide can slow down the production of brown halo. It may require 48 hours for some *C. diphtheriae* strains to produce the characteristic halo. In addition, *C. ulcerans* and *C. pseudodiphtheriticum* may also produce a dark halo on this medium and must be differentiated from *C. diphtheriae*. Other organisms may occasionally grow on Tinsdale agar. *Proteus* produces mucoid colonies and tends to blacken the medium. Rare streptococci and staphylococci can produce dark colonies with a surrounding halo but could be distinguished by performing a Gram stain.

Triple Sugar Iron Agar (TSI)

Purpose

Triple sugar iron agar can be used to determine if a gram-negative rod is a glucose fermenter or nonfermenter, a fundamental characteristic in the initial classification of gram-negative rods. The medium also tests for sucrose/lactose fermentation, gas production during glucose fermentation, and hydrogen sulfide production, all of which are useful in the differentiation of gram-negative rods belonging to the family *Enterobacteriaceae*.

Principle

TSI contains glucose, sucrose, and lactose (fermentable carbohydrates); phenol red (pH indicator); peptone (carbon/nitrogen source); and iron salt plus sodium thiosulfate (sulfur source and hydrogen sulfide indicator). TSI resembles Kligler iron agar except it contains sucrose. Three carbohydrate fermentation patterns are possible:

1. Acid (yellow) butt and alkaline (red) slant indicate that the organism ferments glucose but not lactose. This organism ferments glucose by Embden-Meyerhof pathway to produce organic acids, changing the pH indicator from red to yellow. Once the glucose has been consumed, the organism then breaks down peptones, producing ammonia. This causes a pH rise and reverts the slant to red.

2. Acid (yellow) butt and acid (yellow) slant indicate that the organism ferments both glucose and sucrose or lactose. The organism ferments glucose, producing acid products. Once the glucose is consumed, it ferments sucrose or lactose or both. This fermentation causes the pH in the slant portion to remain acidic.

3. Alkaline (red) butt and alkaline (red) slant indicate that the organism cannot ferment glucose or sucrose or lactose and therefore produces no acidic products. The slant may become more red owing to peptone catabolism.

If there are gas bubbles in the butt, splitting of the medium, or displacement of medium from bottom of tube, the organism is aerogenic—able to produce carbon dioxide and hydrogen gases during fermentation. Failure to do this means that the organism is anaerogenic. Any blackening in the butt indicates that the organism produces hydrogen sulfide gas from thiosulfate. The hydrogen sulfide combines with iron salt to produce ferrous sulfide, a black precipitate.

Formulation

Two formulations (BBL and Difco), available as powdered media, are in common use. Note that the Difco formulation includes yeast and meat extracts and uses ferrous sulfate rather than ferric ammonium citrate.

BBL Formulation.

Peptone	20	g
Sodium chloride	5	g
Lactose	10	g
Sucrose	10	g
Glucose	1	g
Ferrous ammonium sulfate	0.2	g
Sodium thiosulfate	0.2	g
Phenol red	0.25	g
Agar	13	g
Distilled water	1,000	mL
Final pH 7.3		

Difco Formulation.

Bacto peptone	15	g
Proteose peptone	5	g
Beef extract	3	g
Yeast extract	3	g
Sodium chloride	5	g
Lactose	10	g
Sucrose	10	g
Glucose	1	g
Ferrous sulfate	0.2	g
Sodium thiosulfate	0.3	g
Phenol red	0.024	g
Agar	12	g
Distilled water	1,000	mL
Final pH 7.4 ± 0.2		

Preparation and Special Considerations

Ingredients should be mixed with heat and agitation, dispensed into tubes, and autoclaved at 121°C for 15 minutes at 15 lb pressure. Tubes should be cooled in slanted position. For optimal detection of reactions, it is important that butt be deep and approximately the same length as slant. Final medium should be red. Inoculation is done by stabbing the butt with the inoculating needle and streaking the slant using pure culture of isolate. The cap should be slightly loose. If the cap is screwed on too tightly, there is not sufficient air for peptone catabolism. Gram-negative rods able to ferment only glucose may appear as sucrose or lactose fermenters. Reactions should be interpreted at 18 to 24 hours. If read earlier, organisms able to ferment only glucose may appear to be sucrose or lactose fermenters. If read later, sucrose or lactose fermenters may consume the more complex carbohydrates and begin to catabolize peptones, reverting slant to red color. A yellow slant and red butt may indicate failure to stab butt or inoculation of medium with a gram-positive organism. Examination of medium for stab line or performance of Gram stain should clarify this situation. The hydrogen sulfide indicator system in TSI is not as sensitive as the lead acetate method or as that found in other media, such as sulfide indole motility agar. A black butt should be read as acid even though yellow color may be obscured. If hydrogen sulfide is reduced, this indicates that an acid condition does exist and can be assumed. Critical to understanding how this medium works is the fact that glucose is present in much lesser amount than sucrose and lactose. Organisms use the simplest carbohydrate, glucose, first. Once glucose is consumed, they attack the more complex carbohydrate, lactose. If they lack the appropriate enzymes, they move on to protein catabolism. There is sufficient lactose in the medium to prevent breakdown of peptone, provided that it is read at the appropriate time.

Trypticase Soy Agar (TSA)

Purpose

Trypticase soy agar is an all-purpose medium that supports the growth of many organisms. It is frequently used as the basal medium for sheep blood agar plates.

Principle

TSA contains protein as a nutrient source and sodium chloride as an osmotic stabilizer. Agar serves as a solidifying agent.

Formulation

Two commercial products are in common use; formulations are similar in both. The Difco product is called tryptic soy agar; the BBL product is called trypticase soy agar.

Trypticase (pancreatic digest of casein)	15 g
Phytone (papaic digest of soy meal)	5 g
Sodium chloride	5 g
Agar	15 g
Distilled water	1,000 mL
Final pH 7.3	

Preparation and Special Considerations

Mix ingredients in water and heat to boiling. Dispense in tubes if desired. Autoclave at 121°C for 15 minutes. If blood agar is to be prepared, cool to 50°C before adding 5% defibrinated sheep blood agar. In most cases, agar can be added to a broth formulation to produce agar plates. The commercial TSA product, however, does not contain glucose, which makes it suitable for a blood agar base. Adding agar to trypticase soy broth does not accomplish the same thing. Trypticase soy broth contains glucose, a fermentable carbohydrate, which can interfere with the expression of β hemolysis on sheep blood agar plates.

Trypticase Soy Broth (TSB)

Purpose

Trypticase soy broth is an all-purpose medium that supports the rapid growth of most organisms, including streptococci, without added supplements.

Principle

TSB contains trypticase and phytone as protein sources, sodium chloride for osmotic stability, glucose as fermentable carbohydrate, and dipotassium phosphate as buffer.

Formulation

As with TSA, two commercial TSB products are in common use; both have similar formulations. The Difco product is called tryptic soy broth; the BBL product is called trypticase soy broth.

Trypticase (pancreatic digest of casein)	17	g
Phytone (papaic digest of soy meal)	3	g
Sodium chloride	5	g
Dipotassium phosphate	2.5	g
Glucose	2.5	g
Distilled water	1,000	mL
Final pH 7.3		

Preparation and Special Considerations

Mix components in distilled water and heat to boiling. Dispense into tubes. Autoclave at 121°C for 15 minutes.

TSB contains glucose, which when fermented can lower pH. This can cause acid-sensitive organisms, such as *Streptococcus pneumoniae,* to die off at 24 hours' incubation.

Tryptophan Broth (1%)

Purpose

Tryptophan broth is used for performing the indole test, a procedure particularly useful in speciating *Enterobacteriaceae* and in identifying non–glucose-fermenting, gram-negative rods.

Principle

This broth contains trypticase, a peptone rich in tryptophan and sodium chloride that serves as osmotic stabilizer. Some bacteria possess an enzyme system called tryptophanase, which hydrolyzes and deaminates tryptophan to produce indole, pyruvic acid, and ammonia. When Ehrlich or Kovac reagent is added to a tryptophan broth culture, any indole produced by the organism reacts with the aldehyde portion of dimethylaminobenzaldehyde, the primary chemical in these reagents, to form a red color.

Formulation

Trypticase (pancreatic digest of casein)	20 g
Sodium chloride	5 g
Distilled water	1,000 mL
Final pH 7.2	

Preparation and Special Considerations

Mix components in distilled water, heat to boiling, and dispense into tubes. Autoclave at 121°C for 15 minutes.

Inoculate broth and incubate for 24 hours at 35°C. When performing the indole test, the microbiologist should add 5 drops of Kovac reagent to the medium and look for the appearance of a red color in the reagent layer or at the interface of reagent and broth. If Ehrlich reagent is used, add 1 mL of xylene or ether to the broth culture, shake, and then add five drops of the reagent. Kovac reagent is generally used when testing *Enterobacteriaceae* and Ehrlich when testing non–glucose-fermenting, gram-negative rods and anaerobes.

Other media have been used in testing for indole production, including sulfide indole motility agar (SIM), indole nitrate broth, and motility indole ornithine medium (MIO). A spot test employing filter paper saturated with para-dimethylaminocinnamaldehyde reagent has also been used for indole determination.

Urea Agar/Broth

Purpose

Urea media detect an organism's ability to hydrolyze urea. This characteristic is particularly useful in the speciation of *Enterobacteriaceae*.

Principle

Urea in these media is hydrolyzed to form carbon dioxide, water, and ammonia. The ammonia then reacts with components in the medium to form ammonium carbonate. This compound causes a rise in pH, which changes the pH indicator, phenol red, to pink. Both agar and broth formulations do not contain much protein. This prevents the formation of alkaline products from the breakdown of peptones, which could result in false-positive results. The broth formulation contains monopotassium phosphate and disodium phosphate, which make the medium highly buffered. In addition, the broth formulation lacks glucose and peptone. Only organisms such as *Proteus* species, which are strong urease producers and not fastidious, appear positive in this type of medium. The agar formulation is less buffered, so smaller amounts of urease activity can be detected. Also, glucose and peptone are included in these media, which help support growth.

Formulation

Two media are commonly used in the clinical laboratory for urease testing: Christiansen urea agar and Stuart urea broth.

Christiansen urea agar.

Urea agar base, filter-sterilized	100 mL
Agar solution, cooled to 50°C	900 mL
Final pH 6.8	

Component solutions are as follows:

1. Urea agar base

Peptone (pancreatic digest of gelatin)	1	g
Sodium chloride	5	g
Monopotassium phosphate	2	g
D-Glucose	1	g
Urea	20	g
Phenol red	0.012	g
Distilled water	100	mL

2. Agar solution

Agar	15 g
Distilled water	1,000 mL

Stuart urea broth.

Yeast extract	0.1	g
Monopotassium phosphate	9.1	g
Disodium phosphate	9.5	g
Urea	20	g
Phenol red	0.01	g
Distilled water	1,000	mL
Final pH 6.8		

Preparation and Special Considerations

Christiansen urea agar is prepared by mixing urea agar base into water and filter-sterilizing. Mix agar and water, heat to boiling, and autoclave for 15 minutes at 121°C. Cool agar solution to 50°C, and add urea agar base. Dispense into sterile tubes. Cool in slanted position so as to obtain deep butts. Stuart urea agar base is prepared by mixing components in distilled water and filter-sterilizing. Dispense into sterilized tubes, preferably in small amounts.

When using urea agar, streak slant and incubate at 35°C for 18 to 24 hours. If urease is produced, the medium turns pink. Rapid urease producers such as *Proteus* species turn the entire tube pink and may be detectable in a few hours. Slow urease producers such as *Klebsiella* turn only the slant pink. If the organism does not produce urease, there is no color change. Stuart urea broth is incubated at 35°C for 18 to 24 hours. A positive reaction is red color throughout the broth.

Vaginalis Agar (V Agar)

Purpose

V agar is a nonselective, enriched primary plating medium useful in the isolation of *Gardnerella vaginalis*. This organism also produces a distinctive colony, which aids in its recognition in mixed culture.

Principle

V agar is essentially Columbia agar base with added proteose peptone and human blood. The medium contains many protein sources as well as starch, which can be broken down by *Gardnerella*. Human rather than sheep blood must be used in this medium. *G. vaginalis* produces diffuse β hemolysis only on media containing human blood.

Formulation

Columbia Agar Base:

Polypeptone (BBL) or Pantone (Difco)	10 g
Biosate (BBL) or Bitone (Difco)	10 g
Myosate (BBL) (tryptic digest of beef heart)	3 g
Cornstarch	1 g
Sodium chloride	5 g
Agar	13.5 g
Proteose peptone no. 3 (must be added to Columbia agar base)	10 g
Distilled water	1,000 mL
Final pH 7.3 ± 0.2	

Preparation and Special Considerations

Mix components in water and heat until boiling. Autoclave at 121°C for 15 minutes. Cool to 45 to 50°C. Add 50 mL of whole human blood. Pour into plates.

When using V agar, the microbiologist should incubate inoculated plates in carbon dioxide incubator or in a candle jar at 35°C. Plates may be observed at 24 hours, but often 48 to 72 hours are required for *Gardnerella* to grow. The organism produces tiny, dome-shaped colonies surrounded with zones of diffuse hemolysis.

Xylose-Lysine-Deoxycholate Agar (XLD)

Purpose

XLD is a selective differential primary plating medium used to isolate *Salmonella* and *Shigella* from stool and other specimens containing mixed flora. *Salmonella* and *Shigella* produce characteristic colonies on XLD, which aids in their recognition.

Principle

XLD agar contains sodium deoxycholate, which inhibits gram-positive cocci and some normal flora gram-negative rods. Because XLD has a lower concentration of bile salts than other formulations of enteric media, such as SS and HE agars, it is less selective but permits better recovery of *Shigella*. XLD agar contains three fermentable carbohydrates: sucrose and lactose, which are present in excess concentration, and xylose, which is in lower amounts. Phenol red serves as a pH indicator. The amino acid lysine is included to detect lysine decarboxylation. Sodium thiosulfate acts as a sulfur source from which organisms can make hydrogen sulfide. The hydrogen sulfide combines with ferric ammonium citrate to produce ferrous sulfide, a black precipitate. Four types of colonies are produced on XLD agar:

1. Yellow colonies: Organisms such as *E. coli* that ferment the excess carbohydrates produce a great deal of acid and change the pH indicator to yellow. Because there is excess carbohydrate, they do not decarboxylate the lysine even though they may possess lysine decarboxylase. Also, some bacteria ferment xylose only but do not decarboxylate lysine and therefore produce yellow colonies.

2. Yellow colonies with black center: These organisms ferment the excess carbohydrate and also produce hydrogen sulfide. Examples of these organisms would be *Citrobacter* and some *Proteus.*

3. Colorless or red colonies: *Shigella* and *Providencia,* which do not ferment xylose, lactose, or sucrose or produce hydrogen sulfide, would have this appearance.

4. Red colonies with black center: This colony type would be produced by *Salmonella* and *Edwardsiella.* After fermenting xylose to make acid, these organisms decarboxylate lysine to produce cadaverine, an alkaline product.

This causes pH indicator to turn yellow and then to revert to red. Blackening is due to hydrogen sulfide production.

Formulation

Xylose	3.5	g
L-Lysine	5	g
Lactose	7.5	g
Sucrose	7.5	g
Sodium chloride	5	g
Yeast extract	3	g
Phenol red	0.08	g
Sodium deoxycholate	2.5	g
Sodium thiosulfate	6.8	g
Ferric ammonium citrate	0.8	g
Agar	13.5	g
Distilled water	1,000	mL
Final pH 7.4		

Preparation and Special Considerations

Mix ingredients in water and bring to boiling, but do not actually boil. Cool to 50°C, and pour into plates. Cool plates with lids ajar for several hours to remove excess moisture. Do not autoclave this medium and do not overheat. Overheating can cause precipitate formation, which decreases colony size. Shelf-life is 6 to 8 weeks when stored in the refrigerator.

When using XLD agar, the microbiologist should incubate plates at 35°C for 24 hours in ambient air. Some authors have recommended incubating plates up to 48 hours to enhance blackening in *Salmonella* colonies. With any prolonged incubation, the delicate balance of this medium may be altered, and distinguishing normal flora from potential pathogens becomes more difficult. *Shigella dysenteriae* and *Shigella flexneri* may be occasionally inhibited on XLD agar. Some strains of *Salmonella* may fail to produce hydrogen sulfide and, therefore, resemble *Shigella* colonies. On this medium, blackening is more likely to occur when alkaline conditions exist.

Selected Mycology Media and Stains

Patricia K. Hargrave
Shirley Adams

A variety of enrichment and selective media are available to the clinical laboratory in the isolation and identification of pathogenic fungi. This appendix is included to provide the reader with more detailed information about a select number of mycology media cited in the mycology section of this text. Most of the media detailed in this appendix are commercially available in either dehydrated or finished form. Recommendations as to general usage of the media, either enrichment or selective or combinations of each type, are outlined in the mycology section of this text.

Blood Agar With Penicillin and Streptomycin

Blood agar with penicillin and streptomycin is an enrichment-selective agar useful in the isolation of pathogenic yeast and the more fastidious dimorphic fungi from clinical specimens. Sheep blood provides the enrichment, whereas the antibiotic combination inhibits the growth of bacteria.

Formulation and Preparation

Step 1: Basal Medium. Rehydrate commercially available dehydrated brain heart infusion (BHI) agar according to manufacturer's directions. Sterilize by autoclaving (121°C for 15 minutes), and cool to 50°C.

Step 2: Enrichment. After cooling the sterile basal medium to 50°C, add sufficient sheep blood to make a 5 to 6% blood agar.

Step 3: Complete Medium. To each 1,500 mL of blood agar, add 3 mL of a stock penicillin-streptomycin solution containing 10,000 U/mL of penicillin and 10,000 μg/mL of streptomycin.

Birdseed Agar (Modified Staib Agar)

Birdseed agar is an enrichment and differential medium designed for the isolation and preliminary identification of *Cryptococcus neoformans*. The ground seeds of *Guizottia abyssinica* provide enrichment, whereas biphenyl provides a substrate for the detection of phenol oxidase activity. On this medium, *C. neoformans* colonies typically darken to a rich brown as phenol oxidase activity results in the deposition of melanin in yeast cell walls. The colonies of other *Cryptococcus* species and other yeasts remain white.

Formulation and Preparation

Guizottia abyssinica seeds (thistle seeds)	70.0	g
Dextrose	10.0	g
Agar	20.0	g
Creatinine	780	mg
Chloramphenicol	50	mg
Biphenyl	100	mg

Step 1: Preparation of Seed Extract. Grind the 70 g of seed to powder in a blender, add 300 mL of water, and autoclave at 115°C for 10 minutes. After autoclaving, filter through gauze and bring total volume to 1 L.

Step 2: Preparation of Enrichment Agar. Add dextrose, creatinine, the contents of one 50-mg chloramphenicol capsule, and agar to the liter of seed extract. Sterilize by autoclaving (121°C for 15 minutes), and cool to 50°C.

Step 3: Complete Medium. To make the enrichment agar differential, add the 100 mg of biphenyl to 10 mL of 95% ethyl alcohol. Aseptically add the biphenyl-alcohol solution to the sterile, cool enrichment medium: stir; and dispense into sterile Petri plates.

Casein Medium

Casein medium is a differential medium used to demonstrate proteolytic activity by yeast species. Proteolysis is visualized as a clearing of the medium around the inoculum growth.

Formulation and Preparation

Step 1: Skim Milk. Rehydrate 10 g of nonfat powdered milk in 100 mL of distilled/deionized water, and sterilize by autoclaving (121°C for 20 minutes).

Step 2: Agar. Rehydrate 2 g of agar-agar in 100 mL of distilled/deionized water in a 500-mL flask, heat to dissolve, and sterilize by autoclaving (121°C for 20 minutes).

Step 3: Complete Medium. Cool both the milk and the agar solutions to 45°C, and combine the two by pouring the sterile milk solution into the sterile agar solution. Mix and pour the complete medium into sterile Petri dishes. Sterile plated medium should be inoculated by cut streak or point inoculation method. Each run should include the set-up of the unknown and three known controls (*Streptomyces* species, *Nocardia asteroides*, *Nocardia brasiliensis*) using one half of the plate for each organism. Inoculated plates should be incubated at room temperature and observed for proteolysis over a 14-day period. *Streptomyces* species typically hydrolyze the incorporated casein within 2 to 5 days. *N. brasiliensis* typically hydrolyzes casein within 7 to 10 days, whereas *N. asteroides* does not hydrolyze casein.

Corn Meal Agar

Corn meal agar is typically made as any one of three variations on a basal formulation. Each formulation is useful in the cultivation of fungi. Each variation is recommended for the cultivation or enhancement (or both) of particular fungal characteristics. Corn meal agar without added dextrose is recommended for the cultivation of chlamydospore-bearing *Candida albicans* with chlamydospore production further enhanced by the addition of 1% Tween-80. Corn meal agar with 0.2% added dextrose is not recommended for production of chlamydospores. Rather, it favors more luxuriant growth and improves pigment production.

Formulation and Preparation

Corn meal, infusion from	50.0 g
Agar	15.0 g
Distilled/deionized water	1.0 L
Final pH 6.0 ± 0.2	

Rehydrate commercially available dehydrated medium as directed by manufacturer, and heat to boiling to dissolve completely. If Tween-80 is to be added, rehydrate and dissolve completely in 990 mL distilled/deionized water before adding 10 mL of Tween-80. Dispense as 15-mL quantities into screw-cap tubes and sterilize by autoclaving (121°C for 15 minutes). Cool tubed medium, tighten caps, and store refrigerated until needed. As needed, melt two tubes per plate and pour into sterile Petri dishes. Inoculate each plate with a known *C. albicans* control and unknown isolate(s) as single streaks cut deep into the agar or as surface streaks to be covered with a flame-warmed coverslip. Incubate at room temperature, and examine with low-power lens of microscope daily for up to 1 week. Isolates may become positive for chlamydospores (macroconidia) within 48 hours but cannot be considered negative before the fifth day of culture.

Alternate Formulation With Dextrose. Corn meal agar formulation as given here with 2 g dextrose is commercially available in dehydrated form. Rehydrate as directed by manufacturer, and sterilize by autoclaving (121°C for 15 minutes). Inoculate, incubate at room temperature, and observe for growth and pigment production.

Dilute Gelatin Medium (0.4%)

Dilute gelatin medium is a differential medium useful in the differentiation of *Nocardia* species from one another and from *Streptomyces* species based on growth and colonial morphology within this medium. In this medium, *N. asteroides* does not grow or grows poorly with a thin, flaky appearance. Conversely, *N. brasiliensis* grows well, forming compact, rounded colonies. *Streptomyces* species produce poor to good growth with a stringy or flaky morphology.

Formulation and Preparation

Gelatin	400 mg
Distilled/deionized water	100 mL

Dissolve gelatin in water by heating, adjust pH to 7.0, dispense as 5-mL quantities into tubes, cap, and sterilize by autoclaving (121°C for 5 minutes). Cooled, sterile medium should be inoculated with a small fragment of growth from a Sabouraud dextrose agar slant and incubated at room temperature (or 37°C if the suspect strain grows better at 37°). Inoculated tubes should be examined daily for growth for up to 21 to 25 days.

Mycosel/Mycobiotic Agar (Cycloheximide-Chloramphenicol Agar)

Mycosel agar is a selective medium useful in the isolation of pathogenic fungi, both dermatophytes and systemic pathogens. The cycloheximide is useful in suppressing the growth of saprophytic fungi, whereas the chloramphenicol is used to inhibit bacterial contaminants.

Formulation and Preparation

This medium may be prepared by adding 500 mg of cycloheximide (dissolved in 10 mL of acetone), 500 mg of chloramphenicol (dissolved in 10 mL of 95% alcohol), and an additional 5 g of agar in 1 L of Sabouraud dextrose agar. Alternately a dehydrated cycloheximide-chloramphenicol agar is commercially available (mycobiotic agar). Heat the formulation to dissolve, dispense into tubes, and sterilize by autoclaving (121°C for 10 minutes). Place in slanted position to cool.

Potato Dextrose Agar

Potato dextrose agar is a recommended plating medium for cultivation, enumeration, and identification of yeasts and molds from dairy and other food products as well as other specimen types. The potato infusion encourages luxuriant growth and sporulation by fungi.

Formulation and Preparation

Potato, infusion from	200.0 g
Dextrose	20.0 g
Agar	15.0 g
Distilled/deionized water	1.0 L
Final pH 5.6 ± 0.2	

Rehydrate commercially available dehydrated medium according to manufacturer's directions, and heat to boiling to dissolve. If agar slants are desired, dispense as 5-mL quantities into 16×125 mm screw-cap tubes, sterilize by autoclaving (121°C for 15 minutes) with the caps loose, cool in slanted position, and tighten caps. If agar plates are desired, autoclave medium in flask and pour into sterile Petri dishes. Plated medium should be placed in cellophane bags for storage up to 6 weeks at 4°C. Tubed medium may be stored up to 3 months at 4°C.

Note: Potato dextrose agar to be used in the isolation and enumeration of fungi from milk and food should be acidified to pH 3.5 by aseptically adding 10% sterile tartaric acid to the cooled, sterile medium. Do not attempt to reheat this medium once the tartaric acid has been added because hydrolysis of the agar occurs and prevents solidification.

Potato Flakes Agar

Potato flakes agar is used to induce sporulation in fungi.

Formulation and Preparation

Potato flakes (any commercial brand)	20.0 g
Glucose	10.0 g
Agar	15.0 g
Distilled/deionized water	1.0 L

Mix ingredients, heat with gentle stirring to boiling, and sterilize by autoclaving (121°C for 15 minutes). Pour into sterile Petri dishes, and store at 4°C.

Rice Extract Agar

Rice extract agar without additional dextrose is useful in the cultivation of *Candida albicans* with enhancement of chlamydospore production. Rice extract agar with 2% dextrose has been shown to enhance pigment production by *Trichophyton rubrum,* facilitating its differentiation from *Trichophyton mentagrophytes.*

Formulation and Preparation

White rice, extract from	20.0 g
Agar	20.0 g
Distilled/deionized water	1.0 L
Final pH 7.1 ± 0.2	

Rehydrate commercially available dehydrated medium according to manufacturer's instructions, and heat to boiling to dissolve completely. If medium slants are desired, dispense into screw-cap tubes, sterilize by autoclaving (121°C for 15 minutes), and cool sterile tubes in slanted position. If plated medium is desired, autoclave the flask of medium and pour into sterile Petri dishes. Sterile medium should be inoculated by cutting through the agar surface. If the medium inoculated is in plated form, the cut streak should be covered with a flame-warmed coverslip to stimulate chlamydospore production. All cultures should be incubated at room temperature for 18 to 72 hours.

Rice Grains Medium

Rice grains medium is useful in the differentiation of *Microsporum audouinii* from other dermatophytes, especially *Microsporum canis.* On this medium, *M. audouinii* grows poorly and discolors the medium. Other dermatophytes and most other fungi grow well and sporulate on this medium with no discoloration of the medium.

Formulation and Preparation

White rice, unenriched	8.0 g
Distilled/deionized water	25.0 mL

Place rice and water in a 125-mL Erlenmeyer flask, plug with a gauze-wrapped cotton stopper, cover the top of the plugged flask with a paper wrapper, and sterilize by autoclaving (121°C for 15 minutes). Sterile rice grains should be spot-inoculated to prevent confusion in differentiating between discoloration and actual growth.

Sabouraud Dextrose Agar or Broth

Sabouraud dextrose agar and Sabouraud dextrose broth are nutrient media suitable for the cultivation of fungi, especially those associated with cutaneous and mucocutaneous infections. The formulations are identical with the exception of the agar. To make a solid,* plated medium, 1.5 to 2% agar is added to the broth formulation.

Formulation and Preparation

Neopeptone/polypeptone	10.0 g
Dextrose	40.0 g
Agar* (for solid medium)	20.0 g
Final pH 5.6 ± 0.2	

Rehydrate commercially available dehydrated medium according to manufacturer's directions. If slants are to be prepared, dispense into appropriate sized tubes, cap, and sterilize by autoclaving (121°C for 15 minutes). If medium is to be plated, sterilize in the flask by autoclaving (121°C for 15 minutes), and dispense into Petri plates.

Modified Yeast Nitrogen Base—Carbohydrate Assimilation Base

Modified yeast nitrogen base is a synthetic basal medium that provides sufficient sources of nitrogen to support the growth of fungi. Fungal isolates are plated for confluent growth, and carbohydrate disks are dispensed onto the surface to provide the specific carbohydrates for assimilation testing. A dextrose disk serves as the growth control.

Formulation and Preparation

Purified (Nobel or washed) agar	20.0 g
Yeast nitrogen base (commercially available)	0.67 g
Distilled/deionized water	1 L

Mix ingredients and heat gently without boiling to dissolve agar. Once dissolved, dispense 20-mL quantities into 20 × 150 mm screw-cap tubes. Sterilize by autoclaving.

KOH for Wet Preparations

Potassium hydroxide and glycerin solution are used as a mounting fluid in the preparation of wet mounts to visualize fungi in clinical material. Add an equal amount of 10% KOH to the material to be examined on the glass slide. Cover the mixture with a coverslip. Letting the mixture stand at room temperature for 10 minutes or heating gently will allow more rapid breakdown of protein. Examine the preparation for fungal elements.

Formulation and Preparation

Glycerin sufficient to make a 10% solution
KOH crystals sufficient to make the final concentration of 10%

Calcofluor White Stain

The use of calcofluor white stain with 10% KOH enhances visualization of fungi in clinical specimens of skin, hair, and nails. Fungal elements take up the fluorescent dye and, depending on the combination of filters used, appear brilliant green-yellow or blue-white, while the background fluoresces a dim red.

Formulation and Preparation

Calcofluor white M2R	0.10 g
Evans blue	0.05 g
Distilled/deionized water	100 mL

Mix thoroughly. Store at room temperature in a brown bottle. For examination of clinical samples, add one drop of calcofluor white solution with 1 drop of 10% KOH to the specimen on a microscope slide, add a coverslip, and examine using a fluorescent microscope. The microscope used must have either a K532 excitation filter-BG 12 barrier filter or a G-35 excitation filter-LP420 barrier filter combination.

India Ink

The India ink method is useful in demonstrating the presence of a capsule. It is especially recommended for the demonstration of a capsule important to the identification of *Cryptococcus neoformans* in clinical specimens. In this method, the capsule displaces the colloidal carbon particles in the ink; thus the capsule appears as a clear halo around the body of the microorganism.

Procedure

If spinal fluid is to be examined, a loopful or drop may be placed directly onto a clean slide. If cultured material is to be examined, place a loopful of saline, water, or broth on a clean slide. Using an inoculating needle, pick a small amount of growth from a young agar culture, and mix it into the loopful of liquid on the slide. Add a small loopful of India ink, add a coverslip, and examine immediately under the oil-immersion objective.

Lactophenol Cotton Blue

Lactophenol cotton blue is a mounting medium useful in examining clinical materials for fungi. It aids in clearing hyphal elements and preserving fungal materials. It enhances visualization by staining all chitin-containing structures a light blue.

Formulation and Preparation

Phenol crystals	20.0	g
Lactic acid	20	mL
Glycerol	40	mL
Distilled/deionized water	20	mL

Mix and dissolve all ingredients by heating gently over a steam bath. To the dissolved ingredients, add 0.05 g of cotton blue (Poirier's blue) dye. To use, place a small drop onto the fungal material on a slide, add a coverslip, and examine.

Bibliography

Balows A, Hausler W Jr, et al (eds): Manual of Clinical Microbiology, 5th ed. Washington, DC: American Society for Microbiology, 1991.

Baron E, Finegold S: Baily and Scott's Diagnostic Microbiology, 8th ed. St. Louis: CV Mosby, 1990.

Difco Laboratories: Difco MANUAL: Dehydrated Culture Media and Reagents for Microbiology, 10th ed. Detroit: Difco Laboratories, 1985.

Finegold S, Martin W: Diagnostic Microbiology, 6th ed. St. Louis: CV Mosby, 1982.

Howard B, Keiser J, et al: Clinical and Pathogenic Microbiology, 2nd ed. St. Louis: CV Mosby, 1994.

Lennette E, Balows A, et al (eds): Manual of Clinical Microbiology, 3rd ed. Washington, DC: American Society for Microbiology, 1980.

Rohde P, Carski T, et al: BBL Manual of Products and Laboratory Procedures, 5th ed. Cockeysville, MD: Becton, Dickinson and Co, 1968.

Shepard M, Lunceford C: Differential agar medium (A7) for identification of *Ureaplasma urealyticum* (human T mycoplasmas) in primary cultures of clinical material. J Clin Microbiol 3:613, 1976.

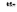